ON CALL
IN THE
ARCTIC

CALL
IN THE
ARCTIC

A DOCTOR'S PURSUIT OF LIFE, LOVE, AND MIRACLES IN THE ALASKAN FRONTIER

THOMAS J. SIMS

PEGASUS BOOKS

NEW YORK LONDON

ON CALL IN THE ARCTIC

Pegasus Books Ltd.
148 W 37th Street, 13th Floor
New York, NY 10018

First Pegasus Books cloth edition September 2018

Interior design by Maria Fernandez

Library of Congress Cataloging-in-Publication Data is available.

ISBN: 978-1-68177-851-8

10 9 8 7 6 5 4 3 2 1

Printed in the United States of America
Distributed by W. W. Norton & Company

To Pat, Chantelle and Adam who shared this adventure with me. And to the memory of Grama Flanagan who would love this book if she could read it now. I love you all.

INTRODUCTION

I decided to become a doctor on a Sunday afternoon. It was the day a family friend, a registered nurse, slipped the eartips of her stethoscope in my ears, its bell on her chest, and for the first time in my life I heard the sounds of a living human heart. I was mesmerized by the rhythmic beats—I counted seventy pulses a minute on my fingers—and captivated by the notion of blood flowing through arteries and veins, giving life to every part of her body. I was ten years old at the time.

Life happened, and when it did, chances of achieving my dream of becoming a doctor seemed to slip away. I was born into a family burdened with addictions and had to accept that the best hope I could have for *my* life was to avoid the path taken by my parents and a brother. Yet, despite odds against it, and by the grace of God, I adapted. I successfully made it through college at a major university, medical school, and an internship to earn my degree.

At the age of twenty-six, on the cusp of launching my dream career as a pediatric surgeon, disaster struck. It was the late sixties and I fell victim to a Vietnam war nobody wanted. With a pregnant wife on the verge of delivery and a two-year-old daughter, I was pulled out of my medical training and buried in the remote, frozen wasteland of Arctic Alaska. There, as a physician with the US Public Health Service, I was left to provide a home for my family and perform feats of medicine and surgery far beyond my level of training or experience.

At first, I was paralyzed with fear. How could I practice medicine in ways I was never trained? How could I hope to be a good father or a good husband after dragging my family to a life so foreign to anything we had ever known? I wanted nothing more than to crawl into a hole and hide.

Necessity and commitment didn't allow me the luxury of slipping away. Overnight, I was forced to adjust to overwhelming need, archaic facilities, and an unbelievably harsh environment. I had to learn to be flexible when my training in conventional medicine failed me; to improvise when medical need demanded far more than I was emotionally and mentally equipped to deliver; and to stick with my instincts and persevere until problems and situations were brought under control.

Be flexible, improvise, and persevere. The actions were familiar; they were those same principles I used to adapt as a child. They would now be the ones that would guide me through these most demanding of times.

Although life and medical practice in the Arctic was severe and unpredictable, it was also filled with laughter and tears. And we adapted to the unforgiving living conditions, impossible medical situations, and perilous travel; Pat to make us a home and me to deliver frontier medicine and surgery far beyond what I ever believed myself capable. For it was never a question of whether or not we *wanted* to do it. It was a question of whether or not we could succeed.

AUTHOR'S NOTE

This is a memoir of my time in Alaska and the life lessons I learned during that adventure. The stories are based on a diary and recorded tapes I kept at the time and are my interpretation of our life and experiences there. In some cases, I have taken literary license by changing names and certain identifying descriptions (such as gender, age, places of residence, family relationships and diagnoses) to preserve anonymity. Reference or similarity to any real persons, either living or deceased, depicted in this memoir or as the result of any changes made is unintentional and purely coincidental. Specifically, no harm is intentionally directed at anyone.

Several phrases and words used in Alaska are specific to life in the far north and frequently differ from those used to indicate the same meaning in the continental United States. For example, except for Hawaii, the remaining forth-eight states in our country outside of Alaska are commonly referred to as the "Lower Forty-Eight" and snow mobiles—such as Arctic Cats and Ski-Doos—are *snowmachines* in Alaska. Muktuk is Eskimo food that consists of frozen whale skin and blubber and an Umiak is an Eskimo boat made of dried reindeer skin stretched across a frame of seasoned wood.

Throughout my memoir, I refer to the many lovely people we lived and worked with in the Arctic as *Eskimo*. Some may believe *Inuit* is a more appropriate term and denoting these people as Eskimo might be insensitive.

During our time in the Arctic the native population was known as "Eskimo." That is how the people referred to themselves then and how they proudly refer to themselves today.

According to the University of Alaska in Fairbanks and the Alaska Native Language Center, most Alaskans prefer the term "Eskimo" because "Inuit" refers only to the Inupiat population of northern Alaska, the Inuit people of Canada, and the Kalaallit people of Greenland. It does not refer to people of Alaska as a whole. Even the word "Inuit" is not of Alaskan origin; it does not come from the Yupik languages of Alaska and Siberia where Eskimo people are believed to have originated.

I would never say, write, or imply anything insensitive or deprecating about Eskimo people, for they are the kindest, sweetest, gentlest people I have ever known.

ON CALL
IN THE
ARCTIC

PART ONE
ADJUSTMENTS

"Happiness comes from some curious
adjustment to life."
—Hugh Walpole

CHAPTER 1

The first time I saw a kid die, he was staring straight into my eyes. I didn't know the boy well, but that didn't matter. My remorse was so intense, my sadness so profound, I knew I could trade places with him at any moment and regret, not a second, the consequences of my decision. It wasn't that I was unfamiliar with death, for as a physician, I'd dealt with it since the moment I made that first slice into my cadaver and inhaled my first whiff of formaldehyde. But I was his physician—his doctor—and watching him lie there, slipping away moment by moment, powerless to do anything for him, tore at my heart until my spirit felt as dead as his.

Even now, recalling that cold Arctic night, to think back on it, to talk about it, is like opening a crypt, seeing again images burned into my mind that time has failed to erase . . .

LATE NOVEMBER, 1971. NOME, ALASKA

I was dead asleep when I first registered the pounding on the door of our government-issued mobile home. Anesthetized in part by the day's travel and in part by the sedation I'd been given in Anchorage for the vasectomy I'd just suffered through, I first thought the racking noise was the onset of a migraine. It wasn't until my wife spoke that I realized someone was hammering on our front door and my night was about to blow apart.

I was in pain. Hours before, I had downed a hefty slug of Crown Royal and two Percodans to ease my misery. I prayed the self-administered cocktail of booze and pills would get me through the night.

"What is it now?" Pat mumbled through chapped lips. "Can't they leave us alone for just one night?"

"Never mind, I'll get it." I whispered. "Go back to sleep."

I sat up in the icy air of our bedroom and cradled my bruised groin in the palm of my hand. *Memo to self: Next time I require surgery—especially on my genitalia—get a second opinion from a physician more dedicated than one pissing away time in the military.*

Our nightstand clock read 2:00 A.M., its radium numbers projecting an eerie glow throughout the trailer's tiny bedroom. The icy chill had frozen our sleeping breath into a fine silvery film that coated the walls and ceiling, encasing us in a palace of crystal. Light from snowmachine headlamps and the occasional passing truck glimmered through ice frozen on our windows and fractured into prisms that decorated the room in delicate shades of reds and blues. It was as if a rainbow had crept into our room during the night.

"God, I wish we had phones here," Pat said. She reached over and pulled me back into bed with her. She snuggled close and draped an arm over my chest. I lay back down and nestled every curve of her body smoothly into mine.

"Yeah, me too," I whispered. I wanted nothing more than to ignore the pounding at the door and drift back into anesthetized slumber. *Probably another drunk wanting something of me,* I thought, *as if the ten to twelve hours I spend in the clinic every day aren't enough.*

The banging continued with greater urgency. Then I heard a familiar voice calling out my name. "Doc Sims . . . Doc Sims . . ."

I clambered out of bed, wrapped myself in a bathrobe, and pulled on slippers. Even the short walk from our room to the front door was brutal in Arctic November without proper cover.

Through the living room window I spotted Gracie Kayuk, my night aide from the hospital. Gracie shivered in her work uniform, her arms folded across her chest. She wasn't wearing a coat.

"Gracie, what the hell? Where in God's name is your parky?" I opened the front door against a blast of Arctic wind and motioned her quickly inside.

"No time for parky, Doc," Gracie said, her voice that stoic Eskimo timbre I'd come to recognize. "Nurse Connie says come quick or kid will die."

"What's happened?"

"Some damn kid be dropped at back door of hospital. Not breathing. Nurse Connie drag him in from cold and lay him on the floor. She doing what she can and tells me to hurry on my snowmachine to come get you. No time for parky. Come quick or kid not goin' to make it."

I rushed back into the bedroom, threw on a pair of jeans and a sweatshirt, and grabbed my winter coat from a hook by the door. I grabbed one of Pat's coats and tossed it to Gracie. "Put this on!" I told her. "This cold can kill ya."

There was no time to explain to Pat why I was leaving. Instead, I hurried out after Gracie. Before I could slam the door closed behind me, a gust blew across the porch and I stumbled on the icy steps. I caught myself before falling, but the jerk of faltering sent a sharp pain down my groin to my vasectomy incisions.

"Shit." I muttered and grabbed myself as I limped down the steps. I felt moisture seep to the front of my jeans, a sure sign that an incision had ripped open. I made a mental note to check it when I had time.

Gracie turned her head away, acting as if she hadn't heard my profanity or seen me grab at my genitals. I was thankful for that.

We climbed on board Gracie's snowmachine and I wrapped my arms tightly around her waist. As we raced to the hospital, Gracie filled me in on what was going on.

"Better make it fast," I hollered over the roar of the snowmachine engine.

The hospital was three miles away and we arrived in less than five minutes.

CHAPTER 2

I can't get a pulse!" nurse Connie Addison cried the moment I burst through the hospital doors.

Connie was on her knees, hovering over a body lying face up on the cracked hospital floor. She was sweating and kept nervously wiping a wisp of blond hair out of her eyes. As I drew closer, I saw that the form lying beneath her petite frame was a young man—a boy, really—white, not Eskimo, with a mop of sandy blond hair. He was splayed out on his back, flaccid like a toy puppet discarded by a spoiled child. His parky had been unzipped and pulled away from his pasty chest. I leaned forward, thinking I recognized him from around town, but unsure. His face, free of adolescent stubble, was sunken and covered with frothy white slime that oozed from his nostrils and mouth. Dried blood stained his lips. A blood pressure cuff and stethoscope lay useless next to him.

"What happened?" I shouted.

"Hell if I know," Connie said.

"What did you get for blood pressure?"

"Forty over zero. Pulse thready."

"Respirations?"

"The wind was blowing so hard I couldn't be sure. If he's breathing at all it's very shallow."

"Any blood stain on his clothes like he's been stabbed or shot?"

Connie shook her head. "I don't know. Don't think so."

I pressed my ear over his nose and mouth, listening for breath sounds. "Pull up his shirt," I ordered. "Quickly!"

I grabbed the stethoscope off the floor, snapped its tips into my ears and laid the bell on the boy's chest. "No heart beat!" I cried. "We need to start CPR!"

We needed help and I turned to Gracie. She was standing tight against the wall, terrified, as if drawing a breath might steal air away from the dying boy.

"Grab the gurney," I said. "We've gotta get him off the floor."

Gracie snapped back to attention and ran down the hall to retrieve a stretcher. The boy was heavier than I expected and as I lifted him, another sharp pain, worse than the first, radiated from my groin. "Goddammit!" I cried.

"You all right?" Connie asked when she spotted me wincing in pain. I hadn't mentioned the vasectomy.

I nodded, quickly forgetting the sting in my scrotum when I noticed the boy's skin had turned an ashen blue. "Let's get going. I'll compress."

Gracie slipped a blanket over the boy's legs as Connie and I positioned ourselves beside him. Gracie made the sign of the cross over her forehead and chest.

I ripped the young man's shirt apart and placed my stacked hands over his chest. I began compressions—one, two, three, four, five—all the way to fifteen. I instructed Connie to breathe deeply into the boy's mouth every fifteen beats. We repeated the rhythmic motion together over and over until the effort exhausted us.

After several minutes I checked for pulses and listened with my stethoscope. I heard a grunting sound, but it was only air that Connie had blown into the boy's stomach.

"Keep going," I told Connie. *What I'd give for a cardiac defibrillator or even a damn ECG in this godforsaken place.*

We tried once more. Again nothing. Then, just as we thought we'd lost him, the boy stirred. He lifted an arm as if to push me away and rolled his head from side to side. His eyelids fluttered.

"My God!" I said to Connie who hadn't seen the boy move. "He's coming around. Hold up a minute."

Connie stopped blowing into the boy's mouth as I stopped chest compressions. I slipped my hands behind his back to help him sit up, confident that breathing would be easier in that position.

The boy followed my lead and struggled to take an upright position. At first he looked confused, disoriented, but then he cocked his head as if he recognized me. His eyes stared directly into mine. His lips parted as though he wanted to tell me something but hadn't the strength to speak. He held the stare for the briefest of moments and then his arm dropped back, his head slumped to one side, and he slipped away.

I silently held the boy in my arms as sadness flooded over me. I burrowed a knuckle deep into his breastbone and rubbed, a maneuver done to elicit a reaction in unconscious patients. There was no response. I glanced over at Connie, my expression telling her that the boy was dead. She began to weep. I wanted to reach out and take her hands, console her, tell her she did a fine job. But I knew the words would be empty. Better just to remain silent.

We looked down at the young man lying still in front of us, mesmerized by the sight. For even when he died, the boy's eyes remained open in a pleading stare.

I had to reach down and pinch them closed.

CHAPTER 3

I never dreamed that frontier medicine could be so difficult. But then again, I never intended to *practice* frontier medicine, so the notion was moot.

Had life gone the way I expected, I would have been sitting in the lounge of my favorite Santa Monica country club, enjoying a Cobb salad and glass of Chardonnay while talking with colleagues about the case of the young man I'd just admitted to ICU for ventilator assistance. After lunch, I'd have summoned my Mercedes from the parking valet, and headed back to my office in a plush, ocean-view high rise to finish out a perfect day.

Fat chance of that ever happening.

Instead, I was bellied up to a smelly bar in Nome, Alaska, called the Board of Trade, hurrying to finish off my second Crown Royal and Seven of the evening so I could order a third. Before heading home, I wanted to unwind from a busy week of medical emergencies and nonstop clinic patients; and spending a little time with my best friend, high-school teacher Garrett Shaw, was just the way to do it.

The rustic Board of Trade tavern—or as locals called it, the BOT—had been carved into the side of an old abandoned Northern Commercial building in the early 1900s, years before the Arctic gold rush had run its course. The bar sat on the edge of the Bering Sea between Front Street and the coastline. It was an eyesore or a landmark, depending on your viewpoint. Air inside the BOT was soiled by cigarette smoke and the smell of spilled beer fused with urine stench that permeated from the "honey bucket" latrine tucked behind the bar. The place was a class A dump, but unbelievably, it was also the *best* of seven bars Nome had to offer.

The BOT was the place locals—both Eskimos and whites—went to get shitfaced drunk and mean.

With my family history and general contempt for anything mind altering, I'm ashamed to admit that I spent many a Friday night at the BOT, hanging out with Garrett to relax the week away. Before coming to Nome I seldom touched alcohol. My father monopolized that little family trait all by himself. But the Arctic has a way of changing things and over the course of my few months there, drinking had become a pastime, a way to get through the bleakness of Nome's treeless landscape and the all-consuming darkness of its winter days.

Snow had fallen relentlessly for five days and it felt good to forget the weather and let go of another hectic week of life and work in Nome. And though it was not unusual for me to be at the BOT before heading home, it *was* unusual to be talking about my work with someone other than my wife, Pat.

"Two weeks ago I had a goddamn kid die from sniffing glue," I told Garrett. "He was only thirteen. He was staring me right in the eyes when he passed."

Garrett shook his head in a gesture of disbelief. "I can't imagine what that must be like," he said. "How do you ever get used to something like that?"

"You don't. I think about it all the time, wondering if I could have done anything more. And the memories it stirred up in my head. Good God!"

"Memories?"

"Bad ones. Things I never wanted to think about again."

"How so?"

"It wasn't the first time I'd gazed into eyes of impending death. It's not something you want to dwell on."

"You wanna talk about it?"

I shook my head. "Right now, I just need another Crown and a few minutes to relax."

Garrett smiled. He understood exactly what I needed and he was there to see that I got it.

He motioned for our waitress to hit us up again, then lifted his glass and clicked it to mine.

"No problem," he said. "Drink up, Doc. I've got all night."

Ten minutes passed in comfortable silence. You know your friendship is solid when you can do that without it feeling awkward.

"Why Nome?" Garrett finally asked. "Did you want to see more of the world before you began your real medical practice?"

I took a breath and allowed my thoughts to drift back less than a year. "Hardly," I laughed. "Actually, it all started with a very unwelcome message I received last April."

SAN JOAQUIN GENERAL HOSPITAL
FRENCH CAMP, CALIFORNIA
SPRING, 1971

It was near the end of my internship and one of the busiest weekends on call since I had started the previous June. I'd had less than two hours of sleep and still faced another six hours of work before I could call it a day. I'd just finished an early morning appendectomy and was in the doctor's locker room changing from my OR scrubs when I heard my name called out.

"You got a telephone call when you were closing," said Denise West, the operating room nurse who had worked with me overnight. "I took a message."

She slipped the folded note between my fingers. "It's from administration," she said with a grimace. "That's never good."

The note summoned me to the office of Dr. David Bernard, Director of Interns and Residents. It felt like I was being sent to the principal's office. I knew of only two other occasions when members of my group had been called to Dr. Bernard's and neither case had turned out well.

❖

Dr. Bernard's office was tucked away in a far corner of an old two-story brick building that had once housed the entire San Joaquin General Hospital facility. The forbidding old structure, with chipped brown plaster walls and a heavy tile roof, stood perched at the top of a grassy knoll, looming over the new hospital campus like a prison tower.

Anxiety trickled from my armpits as I followed signs to Dr. Bernard's office. I entered to the hum of office machines and a typewriter snapping away. A phone was ringing somewhere in a back room. The office was brightly lit, a welcome comparison to the dingy hallway I'd just walked through, and travel posters from places I would probably never visit decorated soiled tan walls.

Fiona McGriff, a fiery henna-dyed redhead from Memphis, stood sentry over Dr. Bernard's office, controlling access to her boss like a mother hen. She was sitting at her desk in the middle of the reception area, sorting through a stack of papers, and did not look up when I entered. I coughed, and she finally peeked above the reading glasses perched near the tip of her nose. She waited for me to speak.

"I just got out of surgery and received this message." I handed Fiona the note. "It sounded important, so I thought I'd best come over right away."

Fiona gave my note a quick glance then tossed it in a nearby trashcan. She picked up her phone and pressed a button. "There's a Dr. Sims here to see you." After a second's pause she added with a snarl, "but he doesn't have an appointment."

I heard muffled conversation on the other end of the line. By the look on her face, Fiona didn't approve of what was being said.

An awkward moment passed. Then Fiona slipped the glasses from her nose and glared at me. "You may go in now but understand this is the last time I'll let you in without an appointment."

Dr. Bernard stood and greeted me with a warm smile. We shook hands and I felt the tension between my shoulder blades relax. Maybe the summons wasn't bad news after all.

"Thanks for coming in so quickly," Bernard said.

I nodded.

"I hear you and your wife are expecting a baby."

"We are."

"Your first?"

"Second. We had a daughter when I was in med school."

"I see. Well congratulations. Now, I have a surgery in about thirty minutes so we'll need to get right down to business."

Get down to business. In a flash, the comment caused my mouth to feel like I'd swallowed a cup of desert sand.

Bernard directed me to take a chair across from his desk as he opened a file folder with my name stenciled across the top. He leaned forward and spoke very deliberately, straining to be certain I caught every word he said. "In the last several weeks have you received any communication from your local draft board?"

I shook my head. "No."

"Where did you register for the draft?"

"In my hometown, South Gate."

"Where is that?"

"A suburb of Los Angeles."

"How were you classified?"

"I was in college so I got a student deferment. After that I got the same deferment for med school then again for my internship. Why do you ask?"

Bernard pulled a paper from the folder and read to himself before speaking. "About two months ago I received a rather worrisome communication from the Selective Service about you. I've been in contact with them ever since."

"Why would my draft board be contacting you?" I asked.

"At first they wanted affirmation you were still in your internship. I assured them you were."

"Have I done something wrong?"

"On the contrary; you're doing just fine. But senseless as it sounds, your draft board has decided to rescind your student deferment, effective immediately. That leaves you susceptible to the draft."

"Susceptible to the draft!" I said. "What in the world does that mean?"

"Exactly what it says." Bernard slowly closed the file and sighed. "It means you may be drafted into the US Army in the next couple of months. Maybe even sooner. If that happens, I was told, chances are very high you'll be sent to Vietnam as a MASH surgeon."

The director's comment was like a kick in the nuts. "I don't understand," I said after trying to fully comprehend what he was telling me. "The deferment I have now should last until I complete my pediatric surgery residency and get started in practice. Can't you . . ."

Bernard cut me off. "You can forget about the residency, that's for sure. They even threatened to take you next month, before the end of your damn internship. I had to pull every string at my disposal just to keep you here through June."

"But why?"

"I have no idea. I've had no similar issues with other interns. And your residency? Obviously, you'll have to put it off until this is settled."

My shoulders slumped, as if every drop of blood had been sucked from my body. It became hard to breathe.

"The way I see it, you have a few options. You can hope for the best, just sit tight and see if you get called in for a preinduction physical. If that happens you can bet the draft is right around the corner."

"And if I don't get called for a physical?"

"That probably means you've made another cut, at least temporarily. You could finish the internship, start your residency, and pray to God you can finish."

"That's quite a gamble," I said.

Bernard nodded. "There is another option. You could volunteer for military service now, circumvent the draft, and maybe get a better assignment. That way there is no gamble. You'd just go in, get it over with, then go ahead with your life once you are discharged."

I paused to catch my breath. "Not much of a choice either way," I said.

"I don't see anything else you can do," Bernard said. He glanced down at his wristwatch, a sign I was being dismissed.

"I'm really sorry, Dr. Sims," Bernard said as he headed for the door. "But I suggest you decide quickly what you want to do. You wait, and the decision will be made for you. That's the last thing you want to happen."

I thanked Bernard for his time. "I guess I better have a serious talk with my wife. It looks like her life is about to change as much as mine."

"Let me call the surgery clinic and tell them you won't be in today," Bernard suggested.

I nodded my head. "Thanks."

Tears were falling before I made it out his door. As I made my way down the hallway from his office, I heard Fiona McGriff call out. "Don't forget to make an appointment next time you come in."

It took every bit of restraint I had to keep from telling her to go fuck herself.

CHAPTER 4

We'd been together long enough that body language spoke more than words.

"Who died?" Pat asked the moment I stepped through the triplex front door. "And you're home early. What's going on?"

"No one died. At least not yet."

"What are you getting at?"

When I finished telling Pat the whole story, she sat in stunned silence. It was something we never could have seen coming. Finally, she spoke. "So, what do we do now?"

"I guess we wait—see if I get called in for a physical."

"Doesn't it help that you're married and have a child and another on the way?"

"Apparently not. Bernard said I'll probably end up in Vietnam treating combat casualties."

"Then you'd be in a war zone. Wouldn't you hate that?"

"I wouldn't like it and I'd hate to be away from you and our kids. I'd hate to not be able to finish my training. But military service is an obligation."

"God, I just can't believe this," Pat muttered. She reached down and cradled her growing abdomen. "I'm seven months pregnant."

My heart sank at the sadness and fear in Pat's eyes. I went over to the sofa and drew her into my arms. With nothing to say that would make her feel better, I simply held her tight and caressed her face and hair with the palm of my hand. We sat together in silence as we tried to let everything sink in.

A week later I was surprised to see Dr. Harry Owens standing at our front door. Harry and I had become friends during the first week of my internship, when he was a second-year surgical resident and I was assigned to his service on my surgery rotation. I liked Harry as both a teacher and a friend.

I invited Harry in and offered him a glass of iced tea. After a few minutes of idle chat, Harry's voice took on a serious tone.

"I'd like to talk to you about your . . . uh . . . situation," Harry said.

"You heard?"

"Who hasn't?"

We both sighed, then Harry began a conversation that blew away the gloom that had settled over our home.

"What if you could fulfill your military obligation in Alaska instead of Vietnam?" Harry asked. "You could take your wife and family with you, and you'd probably have the adventure of a lifetime."

"I think that would be incredible!" I said. "Who wouldn't?"

Harry leaned forward, a wide grin spreading across his face. "Have your wife come in here a moment."

I went to the baby's room and asked Pat to join Harry and me in the living room.

Harry's words seemed too good to be true.

"Do you actually think you could do that for me?" I asked.

Harry nodded. "I just spent the last few years working with the PHS in Alaska. It was one great ride and I made plenty of connections. I think I could put you in touch with the right people to make it happen."

"You'd do that for me?"

"It would be my pleasure. I'd just need to make a few calls."

Harry just sat there, a Cheshire Cat grin on his face. Then he took a sip of tea.

"So . . . when do you think I should start looking into this?" I asked.

"Yesterday," Harry answered. "From what I heard your draft notice could come at any moment. You best make the decision and join the PHS before that happens. You wait, it might be too late."

I turned to Pat. "What do you think?"

Pat smiled and slowly lowered herself into a seat next to Harry.

"Hmm—let me get this straight," she said teasingly. "Instead of Tom going to Vietnam for two years, he could go to Alaska and we could go with him?"

Harry grinned. "In a nutshell."

At that, Pat leaned over and gave Harry a hug so hard it made him blush. Then she smiled and kissed him on the cheek.

CHAPTER 5

My induction into the PHS began with a phone call, set up by Harry, with a Dr. William Hayden in Anchorage. Dr. Hayden was base commander at the hospital and in charge of all commissioned officers. The conversation couldn't have gone any better. As Harry suggested, Dr. Hayden was very interested in the fact that I was considering pediatric surgery as a career choice.

"We are just about to set up a new pediatric wing at the hospital here in Anchorage," Dr. Hayden told me. "We could use someone like you to head it up."

He then went on to describe the proposed new facility and all the benefits it would offer Eskimo and American Indian children from around the state. It sounded exciting, and his suggestion that I could be in charge was irresistible.

If I wanted to proceed, Dr. Hayden said he would initiate the paperwork immediately and I should expect things to move quickly. My internship would end on June 26 and they would want me in Anchorage on July 1.

It was 1971, and hard to believe that in just a few short weeks we could be moving to Alaska.

❖

By the latter part of June, all official papers had been signed and my commission as an officer in the PHS had been confirmed. I was advised of one small change that would happen since my conversation with Dr. Hayden. Instead of being immediately assigned to the Department of Pediatrics in Anchorage as originally planned, I was temporarily going to be placed in Nome. And, instead of working as the head of a new pediatric surgery department at the large Anchorage hospital, I would be designated as a GMO, or general medical officer.

The move from California to Alaska was taking on a life of its own. Time was running short so I meticulously detailed a schedule to insure that nothing would be missed. In the five years Pat and I had been together, through school and my training, we'd moved enough. This time we were going to do right.

First, we were going to need food. Lots of it.

We'd heard that food and household supplies in Nome were scarce and expensive. Harry advised us to buy everything we'd need for an entire year and have it shipped up to Nome by barge. We'd pay for the food, but as a commissioned officer, the government would pay for the shipping. We did our best to calculate our culinary and household needs for twelve months, we got a loan, and bought it all at a big-box store.

Next, there was the issue of transportation in the Arctic.

With the income expected from my upcoming PHS commission, we qualified for a loan and bought a brand new yellow Pontiac station wagon we'd had our eye on. PHS would pay to ship our car, just like the food and personal items, as long as the vehicle went by ground and not air. We only needed to get the Pontiac to Seattle for placement on an Arctic-bound barge and PHS would handle the rest.

Foremost on our minds, of course, was the glaring issue of Pat's upcoming childbirth. Her due date was June 28—smack in between the time my internship ended (along with our health insurance) and the beginning of my commission in the PHS when we would have government health coverage. If Pat went into labor during that no-insurance window and had a hospital delivery, we would suffer financial hardship that would last for years. That meant the prospect of a home delivery was given serious consideration.

Our flight to Anchorage was going to be a major undertaking, mostly because we had a menagerie of pets to consider. Champ, our beagle, was a seasoned traveler. He would be fine flying in cargo. The cat would hiss and growl, but we'd tote her onboard as a carry-on. The parakeet would be carried onboard, confined to a cage half the size of a shoebox that we'd keep covered with a paper sack.

Pat would manage our two-year-old daughter on the plane, the diaper bag, and all the necessities required for travel with a small child. Pat's mom (Grama) would be coming to Nome with us to help with the new baby. We would charge her with managing the cat and bird. I, on the other hand, would be saddled with the biggest challenge of all—carrying the tropical fish.

Pat believed it vital for our children's development they be exposed to movement and color as beautifully displayed in an aquarium. So from the day our daughter, Chantelle, was born, Pat insisted we have a tank of fish in our home.

I was still in medical school, we were dirt poor, and yet Pat's priority was such that we spent far more on an aquarium than we could afford. Over time the Plexiglas tank evolved into a beautiful, serene piece of living art as Pat populated it with natural gravel, colorful coral and plants, and exotic fish native to the brackish waters of the Amazon. She took exceptional pride in the fact that fish in our tank not only survived, but that they thrived to the point of reproduction.

We had a favorite fish—a ruby scat from the estuaries of Brazil. We named him Oscar. Scats are round, flat fish that are difficult to raise and usually dead before they get much larger than a nickel. The majority of scats are green with black spots, but a few rare ones are red and black. That was our Oscar.

Oscar was thriving so well in our aquarium that by the time we were ready to move to Alaska he was larger than a silver dollar. We'd never seen a scat as large. And he was a performer. He would come to the edge of the tank when we tapped and swim around in circles, displaying his beautiful markings for us to admire. He also regularly came to the water's surface at feeding time to have his back gently petted. Oscar was so beautiful, so mesmerizing, when our daughter was just an infant, she would sit in her little carrier for an hour at a time just to stare at him as he made the rounds in his home.

As far as Pat was concerned, Oscar and the rest of the fish were not just pets; they were members of the family. She had no intention of leaving them behind when we moved to Alaska.

I begged Pat to forget the fish, to get serious, and prioritize. She came back with a suggestion that we leave *me* behind instead of them. I might as well have been arguing with the moon as Pat had made her position quite clear. Taking the fish to Alaska was nonnegotiable and as the man of the house, it was my job to figure out how to do it.

I needed to improvise a travel aquarium. It wouldn't be easy, but it wouldn't be impossible either. I just needed a few simple supplies.

I rescued a small old duffle bag from the trash and cleaned it inside and out. For my plan to work it had to pass muster as a regular airplane carry-on. I lined the duffle with a plastic trash bag, filled it with water, and voila, I had a bag of water that would work as a portable fish tank.

I needed a dry run to test my idea, so early the next morning, I went to work. I built the duffle aquarium according to my plan and loaded Oscar and the other fish inside. As soon as Pat climbed out of bed, I showed her what I had done. I was ready to accept praise; she went berserk.

"Are you nuts?" Pat cried. "It will take at least six hours to fly from LA to Anchorage, not counting layovers. The fish will die without air. You can't just tie them up in a bag and hope for the best. You need to have a way to oxygenate them."

Of course, she was right. She was, after all, a UCLA graduate in zoology.

"How about if I keep the electric pump with us and connect it up as soon as we get to Anchorage?" I asked.

"That's fine after we get there," Pat said, "but they'll never make the flight without air. You'll have to think of something better!"

Then it came to me. Where does a thinking man go when there's no place else to turn? Duct tape.

I reinforced the floor of the duffle bag with several strips of tape then placed a second plastic bag inside the first for extra strength. I twisted the opening of the combined bags closed and sealed it tightly with duct tape. No matter how much the bag sloshed during flight it wouldn't leak. I left a small opening in the bag seal through which I threaded a piece of IV tubing I'd lifted from the hospital ER. I lowered one end of the tubing down into the water and left the other end dangling outside the plastic bags and but just inside the zipper of the duffle. The plan was then, when a flight attendant wasn't looking, I would periodically retrieve the end of the tubing from the duffle and blow in several puffs of air. Bubbles from my breath would oxygenate the fish during the hours in flight. Once we landed, I would find a power plug and use an electric pump I'd carry with me in my real carry-on.

Pat listened with intent as I described the plan. When I was finished, she told me my idea was brilliant as long as an overly observant flight attendant didn't spot me and ruin everything.

CHAPTER 6

T he final day of my internship arrived without fanfare. There was hope among the interns that the hospital would throw us a small going-away party, the kind accompanied by a thank-you card complete with a small travel bonus for the slave labor we'd provided the past year. Sadly, there was no indication this was going to happen. The hospital was busy preparing for the chaos the next day would bring when new interns from around the nation would arrive, anxious to begin their year of training. Telling us current interns goodbye was not high on their to-do list.

I spent the last two months of my internship on my OB-GYN rotation. It ended joyfully with the beautiful delivery of twin boys to a couple that had gone through several miscarriages before successfully bringing a pregnancy to term. I congratulated the new mother and shared a hug with the excited father as we celebrated the new lives. It was five o'clock and I wasn't on call. It was hard to believe, but my year was officially over.

I couldn't ignore the touch of nostalgia I felt as I stripped out of my scrubs for the last time. I'd formed strong, caring relationships with many people during my internship year, and I was saying goodbye to wonderful colleagues I would probably never see again. I threw on a pair of jeans and T-shirt and headed for the door when I heard my name called out.

"Hey, Doc," Joyce Brown, charge nurse on the night shift, said. "Come into the nurse's lounge before you take off, will you? You have a couple of charts to sign."

"Sure."

Before the lounge door closed behind me, I was greeted with cheers and applause. A crowd of nurses, aides, ward clerks, and even the housekeeping staff from all three shifts of the OB unit had gathered together to bid me farewell. A decorated banner made from exam room table paper hung over a table stocked with treats. It read: "Good Luck and God Bless" and, on the table next to a cake, sat a large gift-wrapped box.

My very pregnant wife then came out from behind a door, holding our daughter, and joined the celebration. Everyone applauded.

"You and Pat get yourselves over here and dig into this gift," Joyce commanded. "This is something we all decided you needed."

The box was wrapped in colorful blue-and-white paper depicting an Alaska winter scene complete with dog sleds and polar bears. A huge red bow decorated its top. I motioned for Pat to dig in and go to work since she enjoyed tearing into presents as much as any kid I'd ever known.

The box held a large, clear plastic bag filled with items I immediately recognized. It brought a smile to my face. I knew exactly what the gift was all about.

Hospitals are notoriously small, tightknit communities where everyone knows everyone else's business. It was no secret that Pat had nearly lost the pregnancy during its early stages and that we would be heading for Alaska in a few days. They knew her due date lay right in the middle of a four-day gap when we had no health coverage. The gift was their solution to that problem.

The OB nurses had put together a complete home delivery kit. It included *everything* we would need to deliver our baby at home or on an aircraft. The box even included a birth certificate with inkpad for newborn footprints. Tucked in a corner of the plastic bag was a small brown medicine bottle that held one round yellow tablet. I read the label on the bottle and grinned: "Valium 5 mg. Just in case!"

❖

It could not have been a more insightful gift. I was tempted to ask where all the supplies came from, but decided it was better not to know. Then Pat opened the card and read aloud a sweet note signed by everyone: "To our Intern of the Year—Dr. Tom. We will miss you." Inside the card was a crisp, brand-new $100 bill.

CHAPTER 7

The thermometer I'd tacked outside our triplex door topped out at a blistering 114 degrees. The morning air smelled of ozone, a sweet leftover from the electrical storm of the previous night. I prayed for another little sprinkle that morning to cool the air before we got to work, but was out of luck. By seven o'clock the layer of cumulus clouds holding in the previous night's moisture had dissipated, killing all chances of a shower and allowing the late-morning sun to boil the earth below.

We'd hired two men to help with the move. They arrived at 8:15 sharp and started loading everything we owned into a rusted, battered moving van. They were finished two hours later.

"We be leaving now if you don't have anything else," said Ruben Sanchez, owner of the moving van.

We took one last pensive look around the triplex unit, our home for the past year. Anything else we had not loaded in Ruben's van was crammed into the back of our new Pontiac station wagon that, like our year's supply of food, would not catch up to us again for months. We'd carefully prepared our personal belongings for the trip ahead, knowing travel over land and sea could be brutal.

"Tomorrow we move all your things from our van to a sea container and then we'll load your car. After that you'll be hearing from the barge company."

"Please be careful with our belongings," I said to Ruben, "especially our car. It's the first new one we've ever owned."

"You look so worried," Ruben said when I handed him our keys with a nervous hand. "Don't be, amigo. Your stuff will be just fine. I promise."

I thanked him and signed a stack of papers.

Ruben gave our keys to one of his workers, then hoisted himself up into his van's driver's seat. He yanked the creaking door closed, but it failed to catch. It took three more slams before it finally did.

I noticed Ruben failed to put on a seatbelt and I caught myself hoping to God the door would remain shut while he was speeding away with our life's belongings.

"Have a nice trip," Ruben wished us, smiling through teeth that needed attention. Then he turned the key of his truck and the engine belched to life. Black smoke curled into the humid air as the old truck lumbered down the road toward US 99. We sighed as we watched our prized Pontiac follow behind, driven by a man we'd met just two hours before.

We stood silently, sweating in part from the day's heat, but more so from the vision of our life rambling away. Pat reached down and took my hand.

"We are doing the right thing, aren't we?" I asked her.

She nodded and squeezed her hand tightly in mine. "We are," she said. I imagined it was the most reassuring comment she could come up with at the moment.

The truck backfired, lunged slightly to the left, then corrected and eventually headed straight down the road. Just before he turned onto the highway, Ruben's arm flew out the truck's window to shoot us a thumbs-up. It was his reassuring sign that indeed, everything would be OK. After all . . . he had promised.

CHAPTER 8

"Travel is glamorous only in retrospect."
—Paul Theroux

Moving to Alaska was not for the faint of heart. Doing it with a term-pregnant wife the size of a house (her words, not mine), a two-and-a-half-year-old daughter who was the poster child for the "terrible twos," a mother-in-law, a pile of luggage large enough to fill a garage, and a menagerie of pets was totally insane.

We caught a break at Los Angeles International Airport. The loading zone in front of Western Airlines had an opening and our designated driver, Pat's brother-in-law Chuck, pulled right up to the curb. Rain predicted for the day hadn't materialized, so the air was heavy with smog and odors that burned my eyes and made my lungs feel tight. I was looking forward to Alaska where the air was clear, and traffic didn't dictate when you hit the roads.

I hopped out of the pickup and opened Pat's door. She'd been having false labor pains the entire morning and I was anxious to do anything I could to make her more comfortable.

"Get me a damn wheelchair," Pat grumbled. "These contractions are getting worse."

"I think we should take her to an ER," Grama said. "What if she gets on the plane and goes into labor?"

I smiled and thought about the portable delivery kit tucked away in my gear. ERs and hospitals were expensive. We wouldn't be visiting one except as a last resort.

"If that happens I've heard our child gets free air travel the rest of its life," I laughed.

Chuck sighed, Grama frowned, and the bird tweeted.

This had the makings of one hell of a trip.

We checked into our flight with eight huge suitcases and our beagle, that was loaded into a crate for placement into heated cargo. That done, we took seats in the Western Airlines boarding area surrounded by a fort of purses, jackets, children's toys, and carry-ons. Grama sat quietly holding the small sack-covered birdcage on her lap and the kennel with the cat at her side. I kept an eye out for anyone paying attention to us, and when I found it safe, discreetly unzipped the duffle bag, and gave five or six good puffs into the portable water tank. So far, so good.

Pat and Grama made three bathroom runs while we waited. I made one. I was relieved when Pat told me the contractions had finally eased up. Real labor would not have done that.

Our first flight would be to Seattle. After a two-hour layover, we'd board an Alaska Airlines jet for our day's final destination: Anchorage.

After ten minutes, Chantelle began to fuss.

"I think she has a fever," Pat said, lifting her hand from our daughter's forehead. "She has a runny nose and now she's got some sort of rash."

I examined Chantelle's hands and arms. Red, blotchy spots were scattered from her fingertips to her elbows. I checked her legs and face. A few spots there, too.

"Do you have some Infant Tylenol in that diaper bag?" I asked Pat.

She nodded.

"Then give her a dropper full. If she pitches a fit while we're boarding and draws attention we're going to get busted."

Pat nodded. Then as she was struggling to get the Tylenol between our daughter's clinched lips she stopped and leaned forward with gritted teeth.

"Contraction?" I asked.

"Harder than those I had this morning."

"What's going on?" Grama shouted from across the aisle. She rocked the birdcage resting on her lap.

Tweet . . . tweet.

The cat meowed in response.

"Nothing, Grama," I said. "Everything is fine. Just sit tight a minute."

I looked back down at Chantelle. "It may be just a cold, but I can't tell at this point. Lots of childhood viruses start with a runny nose and cough. Many have a rash."

"Will they let us board the plane if she has a rash?" Pat whispered. "Should we ask?"

"I don't know airline rules but I don't think we should ask. We don't want to make something out of nothing."

"Then what should we do?"

"This is Western Airlines announcing Flight 422 to Seattle. Passengers requiring a few extra minutes to board are now asked to report to the boarding gate area."

"That's us!" I said. "Keep her arms covered by her shirt and keep her away from other passengers. Can you handle her by yourself? I've got the duffel with the fish to deal with."

Pat nodded.

"OK. Grama, you ready?"

Grama nodded, gathered up her charges, and we headed for the gate.

Pat looked top heavy waddling down the jet way cuddling Chantelle to her ample chest and protruding belly. I tried to help her while I carried the thirty-pound bag of water and fish in one hand and a backpack over my shoulders. We stumbled twice.

We entered the jet to find a burly flight attendant who did not look pleased.

"Are you all right?" the flight attendant asked Pat after she took one look at us. I prayed she didn't notice the fine film of sweat forming on Pat's brow.

"Just a little tired," Pat said. She shot the flight attendant a forced smile. *Keep smiling, baby. Just get us on this plane.*

"You're not in labor, are you?" the attendant asked suspiciously. She cocked her head to one side as if warning us she was an expert at determining lies. "The airline requires a letter from your obstetrician stating it's OK to fly at this stage of your pregnancy. Do you have such a letter?"

Pat nodded and removed a note she'd remembered to get at her last OB visit. "I certainly do."

The flight attendant scanned the report yet seemed unsatisfied. "Well, I'm no doctor, but in my opinion, you look too far along to be going on any trip."

"Well, my husband *is* a doctor," Pat replied, "and he's here just in case anything happens." With that parting shot, Pat took her letter back and we headed down the aisle towards our seats. Grama followed.

Pat got settled and relaxed with Chantelle resting on her lap. I sat down next to her.

Now, dear God, I prayed. *Just let this plane take off and fly without a hitch. It's been a very long day and I'm not certain I can deal with any more problems.*

CHAPTER 9

My prayer was heard. Chantelle napped, and Pat's false labor pains subsided. For a small woman, Grama did remarkably well juggling all her responsibilities. Nosey flight attendants gave us no grief.

My plan to aerate the portable aquarium went off without a hitch. Every fifteen minutes, under Pat's watchful eye, I reached down and blew ten to twelve deep puffs of air deep into the water to bubble the fish alive.

Our layover in Seattle was uneventful and we boarded the final flight of the day to Anchorage without difficulties.

We touched down in Anchorage around 7:00 P.M. The airport was far more modern, and more crowded, than I expected. Had I not known it was Alaska, it could have been any location of moderate population. We took a cab to the Alaska Native Medical Center (ANMC) on Third Avenue and hired another just to carry our stuff. We got settled for the night in Transient Duty Quarters (TDQ) with a minimum of fuss.

It had been a long, adventuresome day and we were ready for it to end. We hugged Grama goodnight and she slipped into the room next to ours. We finally had a few minutes to ourselves.

"I love you," I said to Pat and kissed her goodnight.

She smiled. "I love you, too."

I switched off the bedside lamp and told her to curl up next to me, as close as she wanted to make her herself comfortable. That's exactly what she did.

The next morning would be the start of a new life.

PART TWO

SUMMER AND THE MIDNIGHT SUN

"And, by the way, I adore you . . .
in frightening, dangerous ways."
—Stephenie Meyer, "Midnight Sun"

CHAPTER 10

P at fell asleep in minutes. I, on the other hand, lay alert, half expecting cries of wolf packs baying at the moon to keep me awake. Instead, I heard traffic noise and the occasional wail of sirens penetrating the night air. It was just like any other city and I felt right at home. Eventually, I drifted off.

After what seemed more like an afternoon nap than a full night's sleep, I was startled awake by a ray of bright sunlight jutting through our bedroom window. My watch read 3:30 A.M., so it made no sense. Then I remembered we weren't in California anymore; we were in the Arctic—the top of the world. Nighttime darkness here during summer lasted very few hours. It was the land of midnight sun.

I crept out of bed so I wouldn't awaken Pat or our daughter, dressed, and went for a walk to check out our new surroundings.

Early morning light, the most beautiful of the day, highlighted the buildings of the ANMC hospital campus in hues of orange and yellow. The sight was so serene yet so powerful it took my breath away. Everything I'd read about Alaska being "America's last frontier" led me to envision the hospital as a sprawling one-story, log-cabin-type outfit surrounded by snow berms and a forest of ice-laden pines. It was nothing of the sort.

The campus consisted of several buildings, none made of logs, and none less modern than any I had worked in. I was most interested in the hospital building itself, as it stood tall and majestic, surrounded on both sides by supporting structures.

I walked inside the hospital and spent the next hour exploring its many wards and services. Surgery and OB units were as up-to-date as any I had trained in. Outpatient clinics covered every medical specialty except pediatrics. I followed a hallway that led me to a modern laboratory and X-ray department.

If this were the type of practice environment I could expect working in Alaska, my decision to join the Public Health Service was right on target. As Harry Owens said: this was going to be one terrific ride.

I returned to the TDQ about 6:30 A.M. and was greeted by a young uniformed man working behind a reception desk. He had razor-short hair and was impeccably groomed.

"Good morning, sir," the young man said. "Identification please." His nametag said *Jackson*.

I hesitated. Damn. I hadn't thought to bring any identification with me when I left the TDQ. I had noticed on my tour of the hospital that everyone was wearing ID and I suspected such was the norm since ANMC was government installation. *Note to self: learn something about government protocol.*

I apologized to Jackson for having no papers and gave him my name. He flipped through a notebook resting on his desk.

"Ah, Captain Sims," the young cadet said, bringing his right hand to his forehead in a perfect salute. "We've been expecting you, sir. Welcome to Anchorage and the Alaska Native Medical Center."

Oh my God, did he call me "captain"? I needed to remember I was actually in the government service now, but it was difficult because everything seemed so . . . normal. I recalled reading in my enlistment documents that all the years summed up in college, medical school, and internship would be applicable to my grade when I entered the Public Health Service. I hoped to God the designation *captain* didn't mean I should know anything about driving boats!

I raised my hand in a feeble salute (I had no idea how to do that properly) and returned Jackson's smile. *Mental note to self again: I really need to learn PHS protocol!*

"Thanks," I said. "I'm just going to go up and see my family now if that's OK."

"Of course it's OK. Before you go I have something for you."

Jackson reached across his desk and handed me a large manila envelope. It was sealed and stamped across the front:

CONFIDENTIAL—FOR US GOVERNMENT WORK ONLY

SEVERE PENALTY FOR PRIVATE USE

I took the envelope, thanked Jackson, and headed up to our room. I felt a tinge of apprehension over all the official protocol, salutes, and government issued documents. It was something I'd have to get used to. Soon.

We passed the day resting up from the previous day's travel. Chantelle's rash continued to spread, but thankfully the Tylenol drops eased her fever and discomfort. Pat had more contractions, but nothing significant enough to suggest true labor.

The instructions given me by Jackson were straightforward. The next day I was to report to the Personnel Office at zero nine hundred hours. The office was located on the main floor of the administration building and I was to enter through the door marked Commissioned Staff and not the door marked Civil Service.

CHAPTER 11

I stayed up most of the night, prepping for my first day as a captain in the US Public Health Service. I read up on government protocol, chains of command, PHS regulations, and proper attire. I didn't have a uniform or business suit, so I had no idea how to dress. I decided on California casual: chino slacks with a button-down shirt and athletic shoes.

I entered the hospital at precisely 8:52 A.M.—or as I'd learned the night before, zero eight fifty-two. The first thing I noticed as I walked through the doors was the stiff atmosphere I hadn't seen the night before. Everyone bustled about without the exchange of friendly chatter and there was a notable lack of smiles on people's faces.

I asked a receptionist the location of Personnel and was directed down a maze of hallways. Near the end, I found what I needed. I took the door marked Commissioned Staff as directed.

A salt-and-pepper-haired woman with lines deeply etched across her cheeks grunted when I walked in. Her name tag read Gladys Boles. She was definitely a no-nonsense woman who reminded me of Fiona McGriff in Dr. Bernard's office.

With no particular greeting, Gladys asked my name and handed me a stack of papers.

"Thomas Sims," I said.

"You got a middle initial to go with that name?"

"J," I answered. "Jack."

Gladys reached in a file cabinet and flipped through some folders. She pulled out one that had my name written on the top tab.

"From now on, when asked for your name, give Thomas J. Sims. That's your name, don't be afraid to use it."

I nodded, but couldn't tell if she was giving me helpful advice or mocking me. I decided the latter was probably the case.

"Rank?"

Oh God, here we go again. "Captain," I muttered.

"You have to speak up," Ms. Boles grumbled. She made a cup of her hand and rudely held it over an ear like an earphone.

"Captain!" I said much louder. "Dr. Thomas J. Sims, captain!" *Is that better, madam? Can you hear me now?*

Ms. Boles wasn't impressed.

"Everyone here's a captain and most are doctors, so don't get your head up your ass because of it," Gladys said. She handed me some papers to sign.

"These forms designate you as an enlisted officer in the US Public Health Service. Raise your right hand."

I did as told.

"Do you swear to uphold the Constitution of the United States and . . . blah blah blah?"

My God, did she actually just say "blah blah blah," or did I imagine it?

"Well, do ya?" Gladys grumbled.

"Er . . . yes," I answered. "I mean . . . I . . . I do."

"Good. Right answer. Now sign here."

Gladys shot me a weak smile revealing two rows of nicotine-stained teeth that looked more like a dried-up ear of corn than teeth. The papers signed, she motioned for me to stand up and leave her office.

As I was about to exit Gladys grunted out, "Oh, I almost forgot." She drew in a deep breath, hacked a couple of times, then said, "Welcome to the US Public Health Service and the great state of Alaska. We hope you enjoy your tour."

I smiled and thanked her.

"Now get yourself on down to Shirley in Housing. I don't want to see your sorry ass in here again till you're discharged."

"Come in and take a seat," a bleached blond named Shirley Harper said as I opened the door to the Housing office. I guessed her age as forty to forty-five, although her dress and makeup suggested she wanted to be much younger.

"Name, please?" Shirley asked, much softer and more receptive than Gladys Boles.

"Captain Thomas J. Sims," I replied, trying hard to sound confident.

Shirley glanced up and shook her head. "My, aren't we formal? You must have just come from Gladys."

I grinned. "How'd you guess?"

"Well we're not all like Gladys so don't worry about her. She's been here since the place opened and her bark is much worse than her bite."

"Thanks for the tip," I said, returning her smile. I could use a friend here and considered giving her a wink but decided against it.

"Now, let's see what I have for you."

Shirley dug through a stack of papers piled on her desk and opened the file. She read, then frowned.

"It looks like we have a bit of a problem with you," Shirley said. "We don't have any quarters lined up for you. Temporary or permanent."

"Quarters? You mean as in a place for us to live in Nome?"

"That's right. It says here PHS has been unable to secure a contract, either private or government, for housing of a PHS physician in Nome. It mentions something about an unauthorized transfer from the Kotzebue Service Unit and funding issues."

I had no idea what the woman was talking about.

"Will you be located in Kotzebue or Nome?"

"Nome, I think, at least temporarily," I answered.

Confused, Shirley asked me to wait in the hall while she made a telephone call. She must not have realized that glass is a very poor sound insulator because I heard every word she said. It was not sounding good.

After a moment Shirley waved me back into her office and asked me to take a seat again.

"My supervisor is looking into something temporary until permanent housing can be arranged. So I'll have to get back to you. Nome isn't exactly an official PHS installation. That's why we have no facilities for you there."

"Nome isn't part of the PHS?" I paused to take in what she was saying. "What does that mean?"

"No, Nome is part of the PHS all right—the Kotzebue Service Unit actually—but everything in Nome is private and not government owned or operated."

If I was supposed to be following this conversation, I had missed the mark. Without doubt, Shirley could see the confusion on my face.

"Look, I'm supposed to send you back to Gladys and she'll take over from here."

"Come on, Miss . . ." I'd forgotten her name and leaned closer to read her name tag. ". . . Harper. Tell me what's going on."

"Well, it's not my department so please don't quote me. But everyone knows about it. Rumor has it some pretty terrible things have happened in Nome recently, so Nome is really topsy-turvy right now."

That *really* did not sound good.

"What do you mean *terrible*?"

Shirley's phone rang and she answered. She asked the person to hold as she waved me out of her office.

"You can find Personnel again OK, can't you?" Shirley hollered after me as I left.

I nodded and closed the door firmly behind me. From a distance I heard her tell me to have a nice day.

"Hello again, Dr. Sims," Gladys said, her voice much gentler than before. "It seems I was a little rough on you earlier. I didn't notice you were the one being sent to Nome."

"Nome seems to be some sort of enigma."

Gladys nodded. "It definitely has turned out that way."

"Care to fill me in?"

Gladys shifted in her seat. "I need to take you to Dr. Hayden. He'll tell you what you're up against."

Gladys ushered me down several corridors to a large office fronted by a beautiful walnut reception desk. A young, nicely dressed Eskimo woman greeted us.

"This is Captain Thomas J. Sims," Gladys introduced me to the receptionist. "He will be stationed in Nome. Dr. Hayden needs to speak with him."

"Does he have an appointment?"

"He doesn't need an appointment; he's with me. Now tell the chief he's here, then go about your business," Gladys said.

It was clear Gladys knew her way around administration. I was glad she seemed to be in my corner now.

The receptionist picked up a phone, spoke a few words, then said, "Dr. Hayden will see you now, Captain Sims. Please go into his office."

Gladys turned to leave, then stopped and took my hand. She slipped her business card into my palm. "You seem like a nice young fella. If you need anything, you know how to reach me."

CHAPTER 12

Although I'd corresponded with Dr. Hayden often by mail and telephone, we'd never met face to face. He was not what I expected. He was very distinguished looking in a military type way, yet he was much younger and less formal than I imagined. He wore civilian clothes rather than a uniform; he was tall and fit, and sported jet-black hair that just touched the top of his ears. He put me at ease immediately.

Dr. Hayden motioned me to a nicely padded chair across from his desk and we chatted for a few minutes. He asked about our trip up from California and how Pat was doing with her pregnancy.

"Still pregnant," I said.

"When is she due?"

"Actually, she's about a week over now. It's driving her nuts."

We both laughed.

Dr. Hayden then opened a folder and took out several papers. He began reading and made a few notes on a yellow pad. Then he turned and faced me.

"There's background on Nome you need to be aware of. It has a lot to do with why we selected *you* for this position."

"You mean *I* was specifically chosen to go to Nome?" I asked.

Dr. Hayden nodded. "You bet you were. I think you'll understand once I fill you in on the details."

I settled back into my chair to listen.

"From a Public Health Service standpoint, the state of Alaska is divided up into large geographic areas called Service Units. Kotzebue, Anchorage, Bethel, Barrow, the Aleutians . . . you get the idea."

Dr. Hayden pulled out a large map of Alaska that clearly showed how the divisions were made.

"There is a modern, well-staffed PHS hospital in each service unit. The Kotzebue Service Unit, the one you'll be part of, is *unique*."

Oh crap, I didn't like the sound of that. Unique is a way of saying *different*. Different often means less than good. Sometimes even shitty. I held my breath, waiting to hear which definition applied to Nome.

"The city of Nome is located about 185 air miles southwest of Kotzebue, yet it's designated as part of the Kotzebue Service Unit. Nome is unique because, even though the town is larger than Kotzebue and there are more Eskimo villages around Nome than Kotzebue, there is no actual PHS facility or government hospital located there."

"And why is that?" I asked.

"I'd deny saying it, but I think the main reason is that Nome has a significant white population. That makes it unlike other areas where PHS provides health services. Last census showed Nome at about 70 percent Eskimo and 30 percent white. It's the whites that run the town."

Dr. Hayden continued. "Many years ago the Methodist Church took over a hospital in Nome, but they could never keep it staffed with physicians. Occasionally doctors would come, usually from the lower forty-eight, but they'd leave after a few months."

"Why was that?"

"Usually because they couldn't stand the weather or tolerate the hostile working environment of the community."

"It was that bad?"

"It was. The native population claimed, during those times the hospital did have a doctor, white residents of town received better and more immediate care than they did."

"Do you think that was true?"

Dr. Hayden nodded. "Probably. And because there were no actual health care services provided for them in Nome, the native people there, who are entitled to PHS care by law, had to be flown up to Kotzebue whenever they needed medical attention. Whites mostly went to Anchorage. It was very unsatisfactory."

"Why didn't the PHS do something about the problem?"

"We tried, but it's very political, especially being so far away from Washington, DC. Plus, there were always racial overtones to contend with. Every time a plan was initiated, something happened that caused it to hit the skids."

"So how does all that relate to me?" By then I was starting to squirm in my seat.

"About a year ago we received a communication from a native group in Nome demanding the PHS provide a permanent doctor in town for the native population. The group had obtained the services of a lawyer in Anchorage who specialized in native affairs, but it wasn't necessary. We had already decided to act on the group's request, but on a local level, without involvement or approval from Washington."

I hesitated to ask, but did. "Was that risky?"

Dr. Hayden nodded. "We tried to keep it under wraps as best we could."

"So, what did you do?"

"Exactly what the group wanted. We directed the head officer in Kotzebue to transfer one of his physicians to Nome."

"Only one?" I asked. "How many physicians are in Kotzebue?"

"Six to nine, depending on the time of year."

"But you planned for only one in Nome?"

Dr. Hayden did not answer.

"What kind of facility is located in Kotzebue?" I asked.

"Everything needed to provide high-quality medical care. There's a modern, well-equipped hospital with full supportive staff including lab, X-ray, nurses, OB, surgery, and full anesthesia."

"So with several doctors in Kotzebue, a modern hospital but a population less than Nome, why was only one physician being transferred? It doesn't make any sense."

"You're right, it doesn't. But none of the Kotzebue docs wanted to leave. Everyone knew about the situation in Nome, and no one wanted to take on the town's drama or heavy workload."

"I can understand that," I said.

"In Kotzebue," Dr. Hayden explained, "life was easy. No one was overworked, and everyone had plenty of time off. In Nome, with only one doctor, that person would work seven days a week and be on call twenty-four hours a day with no help and no breaks."

Crap! He's describing the situation I'm about to enter and I'm starting to get a clear picture of what Gladys and Shirley knew but didn't want to tell me.

"So did you finally get someone who would agree to a transfer?" I asked.

"Yes and no. We got someone, but it had to be by force. Most of the doctors in Kotzebue were Civil Service. Just two were PHS. Civil Service personnel can go whatever they want but doctors in the PHS are Commissioned Corp, like you and me, and thereby obligated to follow orders."

"So if a PHS doc was told to transfer, he would have no choice," I said.

"You're starting to get the point," Dr. Hayden said.

"So what happened?"

"One of the Kotzebue PHS doctors was single. The other was married and had a family. None of the Civil Service docs had any desire to transfer. Finally, the Kotzebue Service Unit Director decided it would be best and easiest to transfer the single person, so that's what he did."

I nodded. "Makes sense."

"It did at the time. Jack—not his real name by the way—was sent, but more or less against his will. He slept in an empty hospital room and ate all his meals at the cafeteria. He held clinic at the hospital but never used the inpatient facility because he had no cases. At first it seemed to work OK, but as it turned out, a problem arose that was huge."

"How so?"

"Rumor has it a few weeks after arriving in Nome, Jack got himself a girlfriend. She was a local Eskimo girl who claimed to be twenty but turned out to be fifteen. Some Eskimo men don't like their women to get tied up with white men, especially at that young age."

"That's understandable," I said.

Dr. Hayden nodded. "Yes, it is, but the situation got much worse. Apparently the girl discovered she was pregnant. Everyone in town thought it was with Jack even though he and the girl denied it."

"Oh my God. So, was he the father?"

"No one knew, but it made no difference. He was found guilty by public opinion."

I felt my eyebrows rise.

"According to chatter around town Jack planned to perform an abortion on the girl and word got out. When the girl's father learned of it, he formed a lynch mob with intentions of hanging Jack naked upside down in the center of town to castrate him. Jack heard what was planned and got a call out to me. He hid out in a shack used by the city as a morgue until I was able to get a National Guard chopper out at midnight to extract him."

"Jesus, God, what a story. How long ago was all that?"

"About four months."

Fuck!

"And the girl?"

"I heard she was sent to Anchorage to live with relatives and have her baby."

"What about Jack?"

"He was transferred to the lower forty-eight."

"Oh my God," I said after pausing to catch a breath. "And you're sending me into the middle of all this?"

Dr. Hayden nodded. "Regardless of what's happened, the town is still entitled to a physician and who better to send than a guy with a family and a baby on the way?"

I paused to let it all sink in.

"I felt you needed to know what happened," Dr. Hayden said. "I know it won't be easy, but at least you'll know what you're up against. Now go back to Housing and Shirley will see what she can do about arranging someplace for you to live."

I nodded and stood to leave his office.

"You have an Arctic survival course tomorrow starting at zero seven hundred hours and ophthalmology training at fourteen hundred. You are then to report for duty at the Nome hospital day after tomorrow, July 4.

The acting hospital administrator, a Mr. Harland McCoy, has been ordered to meet you at the Nome airport and get you to your temporary quarters. Here are your official orders."

Dr. Hayden handed me a stack of papers that I folded and stuffed into my pocket.

"Any questions?"

My head was spinning. Did I have any questions? Ha—what an understatement! I had millions, but at the moment couldn't think of a single one.

As I headed out his door, the base commander offered one final piece of advice: "Watch yourself, Dr. Sims. Do the best you can. That's all we can ask. And hold on to your family jewels. Like Jack, your predecessor, I doubt you're ready to give those puppies up."

CHAPTER 13

I rushed back to the TDQ to give Pat a full account of Dr. Hayden's story. I thought she would faint.

"I get why they selected me," I explained. "They think I'm safe, nonthreatening."

"But what if people find something wrong with *you*? What could happen then?"

"We'll be fine," I said. "I'll find a way to make it work."

Pat sighed and shrugged her shoulders. "You do have a way of getting what you want."

"Meaning what?"

"Meaning exactly what it says. You wanted *me*." She smiled as she made air quotes around the word me. "I'll never forget how you made that happen."

SEPTEMBER 1965
THE ELEVATORS AT THE NEURO PSYCHIATRIC INSTITUTE (NPI)
UCLA CAMPUS, LOS ANGELES, CALIFORNIA

Fall classes had just begun and I was concerned about getting a textbook that was in short supply. The professor said the only location that still had copies was the bookstore at the UCLA Neuro Psychiatric Institute, a short walk from my room in the men's dormitory.

The elevators at NPI were usually filled to capacity ferrying patients, students, and doctors up to the working corridors of the massive institution. I was just about to hit the stairs when I heard an elevator ease to a stop, so I decided to wait and take a ride. To my surprise, only two people were on board: a gorgeous, petite young woman with hair the color of fine mahogany and another woman who I presumed to be her mother. The younger woman wore a short, light blue dress, frilly and modestly cut on top but teasingly high in that seductive space between her hips and knees. She looked familiar and I wondered if she were premed like me.

"You heading to the bookstore to get the book for Comparative Anatomy?" the brunette asked as I stepped into the elevator car. My God, she spoke to me first. I was shocked!

"Yep," I answered. "You?"

"Yes. I hope we can both get one. What if there's only one book left?" the girl teased. "Are you going to be a gentleman and let me have it?"

I grinned at her. "Not on your life. I'm a man headed for med school so the book is mine."

"Hmm," the girl said, hitting me back with a smile. "That's very chauvinistic of you."

"I thought chauvinism was dead." I said.

"Well obviously it isn't. At least when it comes to getting a textbook."

The elevator stopped at a floor and two people stepped in.

I had to think fast. The car would soon be full and this girl was intriguing. "I've got an idea," I said. "If there's only one book left, how about I buy it and we share. Maybe study together."

The girl looked over at her mother and smiled. The mother returned the smile with a tilt of her head that looked approving.

"We'll see," the girl answered with a shrug of perfect shoulders.

"By the way, my name's Tom."

"Pat Flanagan. This is my mother, Vera."

I nodded and shook hands with the mother. Pat Flanagan smiled and extended her hand as well.

I knew in an instant this girl was different; that she was going to mean something significant to me. Problem was, I only had two more floors to make my move . . . and her mother was standing right at her side.

I was never confident in the skills required to deal with girls, but I wasn't about to let this one go. I went out on a limb, took a chance, and before the elevator dinged to stop at our floor, I had Pat's telephone number written in ink on the inside of my left arm.

I called her the next day. We had coffee, dated, and later became lab partners. We sliced apart the organs of sharks and cats and compared how different they were, yet still similar in the way God had put them together.

Pat had the hands of a skilled surgeon and was the best dissector in the class. We both got As in comparative anatomy and we both found our best friends. A few months later we were talking about getting engaged.

❖

Aside from falling in love, I can't admit to really enjoying my college experience. Tight money and my commitment to medical school acceptance precluded the time I could have had for fun. But I didn't mind. I was going to reach my dream of becoming a doctor and Pat was ready to take the journey with me.

When the time was right, I applied to fourteen medical schools. I was sailing through my major in zoology with a 3.8 GPA and I'd done well on the MCAT (Medical College Admission Test). But by mid-April, things were veering off-track. Eleven straight rejections and a provisional acceptance at one wasn't what I had planned.

Toward the end of the month I received a letter from Creighton University. The envelope was thicker than others I had received, and my name was typed directly on the outside instead of on a sticker plastered on with glue. Creighton was my first choice of medical schools and I was surprised I hadn't heard from them yet. Fearful the news would be like all the others, I asked Pat to open the letter with me. She did, and all we needed to read was the opening sentence:

"Dear Mr. Sims. We are pleased to inform you . . ."

Pat and I shared hugs and kisses and then I called my mother. She seemed overjoyed with the news. We laughed, congratulated one another on jobs well done, and made comments about how our prayers were being answered.

But that was when the good news ended.

CHAPTER 14

The two months after I received acceptance at Creighton Medical School flew by at rocket speed. I graduated from college and moved back to Mother's apartment in South Gate, California, to await September and the start of my medical education. I kept the mortuary job I had my last year at ULCA, which was five miles away in Watts, and spent most of my time reading, working, or talking on the phone with Pat. Mother's spirits were high when I first moved home, but shortly thereafter her mood changed. She became sullen and withdrawn, and it worried the hell out of me.

The first actual suicide attempt I remember my mother making was when we lived in Downey, a short drive from South Gate, where I spent my first nine years. I was awakened by screaming sirens and commotion in our front room. I leapt out of bed to see what was happening and, filled with fright, raced to the living room where I found Mother lying on a stretcher with wires connected to her chest that were attached to a machine. I remember her eyes, glazed over and staring at me, pleading. I wondered if she was asking for my help, for forgiveness, or telling me goodbye. And I remember my father cursing in a drunken rage then blowing cigarette smoke in my face, raising a hand to slap me, and asking what I did to make her do it. I was ten years old at the time.

Mother returned home after a month in the hospital and my parents divorced. The courts, watchful for my safety and wellbeing, awarded Mother full custody of me, mostly because of my father's drinking habit and anger issues. I was happy with the custody assignment. I was afraid of my father, his drunken rages and painful accusations, and never once did I complain about missing my dad.

Mother's doctors told me her addiction to Dexedrine, phenobarbital, and Valium was the root of her depression and mental problems. Mother claimed she understood it was the drugs and swore to stop taking them and to never attempt suicide again. I like to think she tried, yet her promise to stop taking the pills was shallow and without merit. It took less than six months for the nasty dragons living in her soul to raise their sordid heads again and take control. I lived my entire childhood hostage to the fear that one day, I would come home from school and find my mother lying in a pool of sweat and vomit, dead by her own hand.

Mother's mood turned dark shortly after I moved home from college and I knew she was in the throes of heavy addiction once again. She tried to hide it, but couldn't. She attempted suicide on two occasions during that time, and after each attempt repeated the same dreadful accusation my father had made years before. She told everyone who would listen it was *me* that drove her to it.

One late afternoon on my way home from work the transmission on the VW Beetle Mother bought for me when I started college failed. I called Pat and she drove twenty miles from her home in Santa Monica to Watts to pick me up and drive me home. It was three hours later than usual when I finally got to Mother's apartment. I entered still holding the keys to the disabled car in my hand, and when I explained to Mother what had happened, she exploded.

"You're a goddamn liar," Mother screamed. She accused me of staying out late to drink and whore with my girlfriend, acting just like my father. She told me I was the biggest disappointed she'd ever had in her life and that I was never going to make anything of myself. She began to cry, then ran into the bathroom and returned to the living room with a handful of drugs. She held out her hand to show me a fist full of Dexedrine and phenobarbital she planned to swallow, and after I knocked them to the floor, she slapped me across the face and dropped to the carpet in a rage I feared might result in a seizure. She screamed and cursed until she tired, then she demanded the keys to the car and ordered me out of her house, telling me never to come back again.

I stood silently, my face burning from the slaps, and cringed as Mother pounded her fists on the floor. I trembled, not knowing what to do or say. I knew it was Mother's mental illness rearing its ugly head again and I should be more understanding. But that particular day, for reasons I couldn't comprehend, I decided I had had my fill.

With no real attempts to ease her pain, I stepped over to Mother's front door and quietly opened it. I would do what she demanded. I would leave her home and never return. I would give her space and time to fight her battles, win or lose, and allow her to live her life the way she wanted.

Rain had fallen the day before, and as I headed down the stairs from the apartment I slipped and fell. I landed at the bottom of the staircase with a twisted ankle and painful back. Gritting my teeth, I managed to pull myself over to a small patch of grass and sat there, sobbing more than I ever had in my entire twenty-one years.

A small balcony off Mother's living room jutted directly out over the grassy patch where I sat. There was a time in the past when I loved that balcony. It was a place where Mother and I would sit, cook up a hamburger or hot dog, and enjoy the evening together. We'd talk about our day, school, work, future plans, anything that people who loved one another shared. Now, in an instant, I knew the goodness of those times was gone forever, drowned and buried by drugs.

A voice called out from above and I thought, perhaps, it was Mother checking to see if I was hurt. I looked up and saw her leaning over the railing, screaming.

"When you leave, take all your crap with you!" Mother shouted. And as she yelled she hoisted several drawers up and over the balcony railing and dumped my clothes and personal belongings down onto the grass below.

I shielded my face from the shower of falling clothes, and when they stopped, I looked back up at Mother, longing to understand. Our eyes met, and I searched for something in her gaze that showed sorrow or remorse. I saw nothing but cold emotion and distain.

A next-door neighbor witnessed the entire spectacle and peeked over the fence separating our properties.

"You poor boy," the neighbor said. "Is there anything I can do for you?" She reached into her apron pocket and handed me a tissue.

"I could use a couple of shopping bags for my things."

She nodded and scurried into her house to return with two large paper sacks from the local grocery. She handed me the bags and I thanked her.

For the next several minutes, I sat on the grass and stuffed my clothes into the paper bags. I was homeless and penniless with everything I owned stuffed into paper sacks I could carry in my arms. All I could think was that I needed a phone so I could call my fiancée and ask for help.

Libby's Donut Shop had been in business at the end of my street for about a year. On occasion, my friends and I would stop in for a snack, but I never had enough money to frequent the shop to recognize anyone who worked there. Chances were slim I could get any help, but I remembered the old saying about any port in a storm and figured, if ever that saying carried any relevance, this would be the day.

I walked up to a drive-through window and tapped on the glass.

"Excuse me," I said to the middle-aged woman who came to the window. Her name tag read Clare. I'd never seen her before.

Clare stared at the sacks of clothing tucked under my arms and I could read her thoughts. Given my appearance, I hoped she wasn't afraid of me.

"I'm not allowed to serve you at the drive up," Clare said. "Come around to the walk-up window in front."

The sweet aromas of fried bread and glaze whiffed up from inside the shop as Clare slid open a glass window, but I was hurting too much for the smells to interest me. Clare asked me what I wanted to order and I shook my head.

"I don't want a doughnut, thank you," I said. "What I really need is some help. I don't have any money, but I need to make a long-distance phone call to Santa Monica. Could I use your phone? I promise I'll pay you back."

Clare shook her head. "I'm sorry but I'm not allowed to let customers use the phone."

It was getting dark and I needed a place to sleep for the night. I felt panic about to set in. I thought a moment.

"You said you're not allowed to let *customers* use the phone," I said. "But since I don't have any money to buy anything, technically I'm not a customer. Please . . ." I pleaded with her. "I really am desperate."

Clare looked around the shop. There were no other customers inside or at the service windows. "Well aren't you the clever young man," she said with a warm smile. "You're right, you're not a customer. So, I don't see where there's any problem. Come around to the back door and I'll let you in. But don't touch anything. I'll bring you the phone."

I walked to the back of the shop and Clare ushered me in. She motioned for me to sit on a stool next to a big stainless-steel table that was dusty with white flour. She brought me the phone and, along with it, a chocolate doughnut and a cup of milk. She set the treats on the table and turned away to give me privacy.

Pat cried when I told her what happened. When she settled down I asked if she could come get me. She told me to hold the phone. After a couple of minutes, she came back on.

"I asked Mom and she said you could stay here as long as you like," Pat said. "I'll make up a room for you and my brother-in-law, Chuck, will come pick you up."

I finished the call and started out the door. "Thank you so much," I hollered to Clare who was at the front of the shop finishing up with a customer. "I don't know when, but I will pay you back."

Clare turned and came back toward me and smiled. "You needn't worry about the call. I'm glad I could help."

I was glad she could help too, but for reasons more than merely loaning me the phone. I needed to see there was still good in the world. My neighbor and Clare helped me realize that.

I finished the doughnut then crossed the street to sit on the curb and wait for Chuck. I sulked, feeling angry, afraid, and alone. I hurt in such a way a part of me simply wanted to fade away into the night and forget.

The conversation I had with Pat was the hardest call I'd ever made; yet the doughnut was the sweetest I'd ever tasted.

CHAPTER 15

Two agonizing hours passed. Santa Monica was just an hour away, so I began to worry that perhaps Pat was having second thoughts about our relationship. Maybe she was starting to feel I wasn't worth the effort now that my life had drastically changed.

Finally, a blue pickup I recognized pulled up to the curb and I put my concerns away.

"Sorry I'm so late," Chuck said through his driver's window. "Traffic was a bear and I got lost trying to find you."

"It's OK. I'm just glad you're here."

"I hear things have pretty much gone south."

I nodded. "That's one way to put it."

"Well climb in and I'll take you to Santa Monica. I think things will be better there."

I got in the truck and pulled the door shut. "Thanks again for coming."

"Glad I could help," Chuck said.

His comment reminded me of Clare. "Hold on a second. Do you have five bucks you can loan me?" I asked.

Chuck pulled out his wallet and withdrew a bill. It was a five. "Is this enough?"

"I think so. I'll be right back."

I jumped out of the truck and walked over to the doughnut shop window. Clare spotted me and opened up.

"Still here?" she asked. "You need to make another call?"

I shook my head. "No, someone's here to get me."

Then I reached across the counter and handed Clare the five-dollar bill. "I hope this will cover the call and the milk and doughnut."

Clare smiled as she took the bill and turned it over in her weathered hand.

"You hang onto this," she said as she placed the bill onto the counter and slid it back towards me.

"But I owe for the food and the phone call."

"Don't even think about it. I've already taken care of the snack. It was just a doughnut and a glass of milk. And I think the company can afford the call."

It was hard to know what to say. I picked up the bill to give back to Chuck.

"Thank you," I said. "You've been more than kind to me."

As I was getting ready to leave, Clare smiled softly and reached across the counter to take my hand in hers. "You know, it's none of my business," she said, "but you seem like a nice young man. I don't know what your trouble is, but you have my prayers."

My call to Creighton Medical School the next day was answered by the secretary to the dean. When I told her I had to release my acceptance to school, she connected me to Father Quinn, head of the medical school and higher in authority than even her boss. Embarrassed and humiliated about my family life, I minimized my reasons for dropping from the class, sticking simply to the fact my financial support had disappeared and I had no money to attend school.

I don't think Father Quinn was fooled. The tone of his voice said he knew more of my situation than I was willing to disclose.

"I have your application in front of me right now," the priest said. "You did very well in college and on the MCAT examination. And I must say you certainly impressed our alumnus, Dr. Wilson, who conducted your personal interview. He said you would be a credit to Creighton and a credit to the medical community."

"Thank you," I was able to get out.

"We take that to heart," Father Quinn said, "and at Creighton we don't admit students based upon their ability to pay."

The conversation paused. "Do you have a way to get to Omaha right away?" the priest asked.

Pat and I had stayed up all night talking about what we were going to do. Pat's sister and her husband offered a loan of $1500, if I thought that might help.

"I think I can come up with something."

"Good. If not, we'll send you a plane ticket. If you will work summer session in the cafeteria slinging hash, we'll give you meals and a room in the dorm. Once your classes start, we'll figure out the next step."

I couldn't believe Father Quinn's words. The next day I bought the cheapest flight I could find to Omaha and three days later I was on my way to the rest of my life.

We decided Pat would continue at UCLA one more quarter to complete her bachelor of arts degree in zoology. Three months later, on Christmas Day, 1966, she boarded a plane and joined me. It took less than a week for her to secure a job as a clinical researcher at the Nebraska Psychiatric Institute. The following June, we returned to Santa Monica for a quick trip home in order to be married.

CHAPTER 16

T he bright, early morning sun pouring through the window made it easy to bounce out of bed, get fed, dressed, and off to the hospital for my Arctic training course at zero seven hundred hours.

Arctic survival training sounded important, but it turned out to be a joke. I learned only three things: how to build an igloo using my bare hands should I be involved in a winter plane crash; the importance of walking in circles if caught in an unexpected whiteout; and how to cover myself with mud in a summer plane crash so mosquitos wouldn't finish me off (if the crash didn't). My ophthalmology training was even worse. I learned I would need to perform eye refractions and fit glasses when I went out on village visits. When I told my trainer I had no experience in eye work, he told me it wouldn't be a problem. The best way to help people find glasses was to let them choose the glasses themselves from a box.

While I was occupied with "training," Pat followed the advice of a PHS wife she met at the TDQ and visited a local market to pick up a few basics for taking on the plane. The items would tide us over until she could go shopping for real. By nightfall, we were ready to hit the bed in preparation for the next day when, at zero nine hundred hours, we would board a flight to our new Arctic home.

Everyone on the plane was loaded down with carry-ons, so no one paid any attention to us and all of our garb. Life was difficult in the Arctic, and every time people from the bush traveled to Anchorage, they loaded up on things not available locally and toted them back home on the jet. The airlines knew all about the practice but turned their heads the other way.

The flight was smooth, and our jet touched town on the asphalt of the Nome airfield in little over an hour and a half.

From the moment I first saw him, I knew Mr. Harlan McCoy was not a man to be trusted. He had beady eyes that shifted with every word he spoke and a toothy smile that looked forced and insincere. My suspicions were verified by the first few words he spoke.

"Dr. Sims, I presume," the wiry, balding man said as he watched us lug our mass of carry-ons into the Nome terminal. He made no offer to help. "My name is Mr. McCoy. I've been asked by someone at the Anchorage hospital to meet you and show you to your temporary quarters."

"I'm Tom Sims," I said, extending my hand and introducing Pat, Grama, and Chantelle.

McCoy shook my hand with a grip so weak it sent a chill down my spine.

"Pleased to meet you," he muttered as if he wasn't.

"Are you with the PHS?" I asked.

"Goodness, no. I'm the acting administrator of the Maynard McDougall Hospital where you'll be working. Our permanent administrator is in the lower forty-eight on business. I'm meeting you strictly as a favor to . . . someone. I don't recall the name."

"I see, well thank you for meeting us."

McCoy nodded. "Your temporary housing is a small bungalow owned by the BIA—Bureau of Indian Affairs. It's about ten miles out of town. Are you waiting for any more bags? I'd really like to get back to the hospital."

"Several."

"I see. Well, perhaps you can round up someone to help you. It appears your tired wife and older mother-in-law won't be much assistance."

I felt the hair on my neck bristle at his rude comment. "We'll manage," I said, wondering what the hell was up with the guy.

"I'm also supposed to present you with your temporary transportation."

"I wasn't aware I would be given transportation," I said. "That's good news."

"Don't get your hopes up. It isn't much. And don't expect me to explain anything further as I know nothing more. Your permanent housing arrangements or transportation needs are none of my concern."

"I understand," I said. "And you don't have to wait until our bags are unloaded. Just show me to my transportation and I'll take it from there."

McCoy nodded. "Very well. Follow me."

McCoy led me to a gravel parking area just outside the terminal building where sat a classic World War II Jeep field ambulance that looked like it had been pulled out of the movies. He nodded towards the vehicle.

"The keys are in the ignition," McCoy said. "It's rough riding, but it will get you where you need to go." He added with a chuckle, "As if there were any places *to* go."

McCoy seemed to think the ambulance would appall me, but I was actually delighted. The drab military green truck sported two clunky side doors plus a double-wide cargo door at the rear. Huge red crosses decorated both sides. Inside was a stock driver's chair and a makeshift passenger seat someone had fashioned from a folding chair secured to the floorboard by hooks and wires. There were no rear seats, shelves, or anything else to fill a huge, wide-open cargo space in back. It was just what we needed to haul all our gear.

I hopped in the Jeep, turned the key, and was thrilled when black smoke burped from the tail pipe as the engine roared to life.

As I was showing Pat and Grama the Jeep, I saw McCoy climb into a tiny white Datsun truck and start its engine. Then, just as he was about to leave, he turned the truck around and approached me.

"The envelope on the dash contains a map to your house. But be aware, the house is reserved for BIA teachers so don't get too comfortable. You will have to move out immediately when they return."

"When will that be?"

"In about three weeks," McCoy said with an obvious smirk.

I frowned. "Then where will we live?"

McCoy got out of his truck and walked over to the ambulance. "As I said before Dr. Sims, your housing requirements are none of my concern. I had to go out of my way just to locate this temporary place for you, but don't expect anything more from me."

"OK," I said. "Sorry."

"It's important you remember this: I don't work for you or the Public Health Service. In fact, truth be told, *you* work for me." He accentuated each word with a finger point. I resisted the temptation to grab the finger and bend it till it snapped.

So he thought I worked for him. Ha! That was something I would have to get straightened out very quickly.

We piled our gear into the back of the ambulance and, following McCoy's map, bounced our way over a heavily rutted road out to the BIA house. Pat sat on the makeshift passenger seat with Chantelle on her lap and suffered false labor pains while Grama jostled around the cargo area with our luggage and animals.

The BIA house was a one-bedroom, pink clapboard shack built right across the road from the Bering Sea. It was built on sand and tundra and was elevated on stilts to protect against flooding. Furnishings, as such, included a small sofa and chair in the main living room, a tiny kitchen with a two-burner stove, a refrigerator, and a smattering of drawers and cabinets. The bedroom had a double bed that looked as if it were army surplus, much like the vintage ambulance we'd been given to use.

Fortunately, the house did have running water that we soon determined was pumped from a large storage tank inside the house. We had heat from an oil-burning stove and remarkably, electricity. We soon heard those utilities were more than many homes in town could boast so we felt blessed. It was Grama who discovered the commode.

"Come look at this!" Grama hollered.

The toilet looked more like it belonged in an outhouse than anything I'd ever seen inside a home. A conventional toilet seat was bolted down to a piece of plywood and seated atop a wooden box about one-foot square. There was no actual toilet, per se: no tank, no flushing mechanism. The lid of the toilet seat was down.

Though not terribly anxious to do so, I lifted the toilet seat up to investigate and was struck by an indescribable odor. I peered inside, but, thank God, it was too dark to see anything.

"Far as I can tell, it's OK," I told Grama. "Go ahead and use it."

I closed the door and went into the bedroom to unpack.

Moments later I heard Grama shriek and raced back to bathroom to catch her bolting out of the toilet, frantically pulling up her underwear and convulsing with laughter.

"What happened?" I shouted.

Grama's face was beet red. "I was sitting on the toilet when all of a sudden I heard a door open directly under me. A cold wind blew right up my bottom and then I heard this scraping noise. I screamed and distinctly heard someone say 'Sorry, ma'am.' It scared the living daylights out of me."

I dashed out the front door to see what was going on. There, parked right in front of the house, was a large tanker truck with a sign written on the side: Nome Honey Bucket Service.

An Eskimo man with a frown on his face looked over at me and shouted, "So sorry, sir. Didn't know anyone be sitting on da pot. Happens every now and den."

"What is this?" I asked.

"You must be new to Nome."

I introduced myself and told him we'd just arrived.

"Most houses in Nome have honey buckets 'cause we got no sewers like you probably used to in lower forty-eight. Here, when you . . . er . . . have to go to bat'room, it collects in dese pots called honey buckets and I'm da guy who changes buckets for you. I come bout three o' four times inna week and grab da pot from outside da house through little doors. Sorry to do it when wife be using da pot."

I grinned and explained it was my mother-in-law and not my wife on the toilet and we both shrugged. He apologized again.

"Thanks for telling me about this," I said. "I've never heard of honey buckets and I'll tell the others in my family."

"Good idea you do dat. Mother-in-law nearly give me a heart attack when I open door to get bucket and she scream. I t'ink she scare me just bout as much as I scare her."

With the Bering Sea right outside our living room window, there was no containing Grama's excitement. Grama wasn't about to let anything stand in the way of our ocean view so, soon after she settled down from the honey bucket incident, she went to work. She gathered up a wad of discarded newspapers and leftover paper towels she found in a cupboard and, using just water and spit, went outside and scrubbed away months of salt and dirt that had collected on the windows since the teachers had left the previous May. The fruit of her labor was spectacular.

Gone were the high-rises and condos that dotted the shoreline of the Santa Monica coast. Gone were the highways, the traffic I loathed, the beachgoers scrambling for a place to park. There were no ships, no oil rigs, not a single pleasure boat as far as the eye could see. The only obstacle that disrupted the beauty of the quiet horizon was the glimmering summer sun as it made its arc across the open ocean in front of us. There was complete silence, broken only by the blow of an occasional whale or the lapping of tiny waves upon the sandy shoreline. It was sky, earth, and sea in its natural state, the way it had been since the beginning of time.

CHAPTER 17

"There's no place like Nome."
—Town motto

We were starved. My plan to drop into a Nome café for some lunch on the way to the BIA house fell flat. There were no cafés in Nome. Neither was there a convenience market nor a fast-food joint where we could grab a burger.

It was now time for dinner and all we had were the few staples Pat had picked up before we left Anchorage. Our barge with supplies wouldn't arrive for several more weeks and getting food and mere basics was going to take some creative thinking.

In just an afternoon we had learned three important facts about life in the Arctic: we'd be using a toilet that could literally be pulled out from under us; we would need food and should seize every opportunity to get some; and we'd best be careful how we used our water since it was stored in tanks and would constantly be in short supply.

"Let's go to town and explore," I said. "Maybe we can find a place to grab some supper and we could use a little break from the house."

No one objected, so we piled into the ambulance and headed out for our first adventure into our new community.

It was like the ambulance was a time machine that had landed us back in the 1800s. Our first impression was that Nome was a shantytown; a settlement of tiny houses built of plywood and corrugated metal, lined up door to door on streets made of matted down dirt and gravel. There was no landscaping around the houses because there were no yards to accommodate landscaping. There were no services such as water or sewers, streetlights, telephones, curbs, or sidewalks, and nothing to give the town personality. Everything was built from a functional standpoint to get through the brutal harshness of winter. Survival was the only concern; aesthetics mattered little.

Front Street, the only commercial avenue in town, bordered the shoreline of the Bering Sea. It ran from the far west end of town about twenty miles east, past the BIA house and on to a restaurant called The Roadhouse. Front was the only paved road in town. It was unlined, rugged, and besieged by frost-fractured potholes and fissures. In the middle of town and on the seaward side, Front Street was lined by an old-fashioned wooden boardwalk.

Several vehicles—mostly bruised, rusted-out pickups—were parked against the wooden walk that ran along Front Street's edge. Three businesses on the street comprised the major portion of Nome's business district.

First was the Board of Trade tavern. Just down the block stood a stately hotel called the Golden Nugget Inn. Between the BOT and the "Nugget" was a general store, the NC—short for Northern Commercial. Across the street and down half a block rose the glimmering marquee of a movie theater, cleverly called the Nomerama.

We parked the ambulance in front of the Golden Nugget Inn and went inside. I felt certain there would be a restaurant where we could get a meal. I was partly right. They did have a restaurant, but it operated only on Friday and Saturday nights. Today it was closed.

Our visit to the Nugget was not without benefit. We learned that Alaska Airlines owned the hotel and on Friday nights, when weather conditions permitted their plane to land, the hotel offered a buffet that featured fresh salads and fried shrimp. Salad would become one of the many food items we would miss in Nome. We would patronize the buffet as often as we could afford the outrageous five dollars per plate price the hotel charged. It wouldn't be often.

The NC sold plenty: breakup boots, jackets and shirts, fishing and hunting goods, and a few groceries. Glaringly missing from its shelves were fresh milk, cheese, eggs, and meat. Like everything else in town, the NC was closed on Sundays and holidays, and it was ghastly expensive. But it was the only place we could get supplies until we found out how to order things from Anchorage or until our barge arrived from Seattle.

My enthusiasm for the next day—my first as a bush doctor in the Arctic—was dampened by hunger and fatigue. Pat and I had spent a restless night: she suffering false labor pains and me sympathizing right along with her.

I'd been anxious to see the Maynard McDougall Memorial Hospital ever since learning its history from Dr. Hayden and meeting its colorful administrator, Mr. Harlan McCoy. I could only imagine what obstacles I would face there, given the stories I'd been told. I hoped the residents of Nome and surrounding villages would give me a chance to prove myself before judging me based upon the ill-chosen actions of my predecessor.

At 7:00 A.M. Monday morning I fired up the ambulance and headed off to the hospital. It took thirty minutes to travel the ten miles over gravel and pothole-laden streets in a broken-down Jeep that had had no service or shock work since the 1940s.

My first look at the hospital gave me pause, for it resembled more the façade of a mental institution I'd seen in movies than a health care facility. Painted a dark, moldy green, the place looked as if it hadn't had a coat of paint or a facelift since it was built in 1906. Had there been a chain-link fence surrounding its borders and a tower at each corner, it would have passed as a prison.

The lobby was stark and empty of people. A dozen plastic chairs lined a wall of chipped plaster, soiled by years of body sweat and cigarette smoke. A musty odor of age and the acrid smell of disinfectant hung in the air. A reception desk, currently unmanned and marked CLINIC CHECK-IN, was set off to one side of the seating area. There was a door at the opposite end of the lobby that was marked CLINIC ENTRANCE. I checked the door. Locked.

To the right of the lobby lay a dimly lit hallway that led to an inpatient area. I had barely begun to explore when I was approached by a young, fair-haired nurse wearing a starched white uniform, white stockings, and white shoes. She was tall, thin as a rail, and had a pleasant face free of makeup. Wispy hair hung in unkempt ringlets around the edges of her nurse's cap.

"May I help you?" the nurse asked. Her name tag read Sally R.

"My name is Tom Sims . . . Dr. Sims, actually," I said. "I'm the new PHS doc starting today."

Nurse Sally's face brightened into a wide smile. "Dr. Sims, we have been expecting you." She extended a hand and we shook vigorously. "I'm so glad to meet you."

"Same here," I said. She had a firm grip that I liked.

"I'm Sally Reynolds, Director of Nurses—for whatever that's worth." She chuckled, and I joined in the laugh.

I looked around the hallway and poked my head into a patient room. It was ancient. A bed sat in the center of the room with an empty chart dangling from its foot rail. There was no TV, no ports in the wall for oxygen, and not even a nurse call button.

"So this is Maynard McDougall Memorial Hospital. I've heard a lot about her."

"And not all good," Sally teased, "but we try our best. Actually her official name is Maynard McDougall Methodist Memorial Hospital, but that's a mouthful so we usually just call her the MMM."

"Makes sense."

"Sometimes, depending upon how many beers we've had at the BOT, we call her the Maynard McDougall Mausoleum."

"Ouch!" I exclaimed. "That doesn't sound good."

Sally shrugged.

"Care to explain?" I said.

"I imagine you've heard about the happenings with our last doctor," Sally said it with a flinch that suggested the topic was still a thorn to be reckoned with, and preferably avoided.

I nodded. "Everyone's referred to him as Jack."

"Right. Well . . . Jack left about four months ago. Escaped, you might say."

"So, you've been without a doctor that long?"

"Essentially. There's been a doctor that drops in from Kotzebue for a day or so every now and then, but it's not nearly enough. I'm sure you've heard there's a bit of animosity between the hospital administration and the PHS."

"I have. What's with that?"

"I think it's because administration resents the fact they have to depend on the PHS to fill the place with a doctor."

"So how does the hospital get nurses like you? Are you PHS?"

"No. With us, it's a little different. We're actually part of a Catholic mission here in Nome that supports a radio station called KNOM. We broadcast contemporary music throughout Nome and all the villages on the peninsula. But instead of having regular commercials, we send out health tips and community messages."

Music and health. Not a bad combination.

"All the nurses live in a dorm at the station and donate our salaries in return for room and board. All our DJs are aspiring disc jockeys who are donating their time for experience."

"That sounds really great," I said. "I hope to meet everyone associated with the station."

"Oh, don't worry, you will. Our director, Father James Poole, has big plans for you. It won't be long before he'll have you writing and recording health spots."

I grinned. "We'll see."

"You don't know Father Poole. He's very persuasive."

Sally then directed me toward a set of double doors marked Operating Room. She was about to step inside when I stopped her.

"Shouldn't we change into scrubs before going in? Sterile precautions."

"I don't know why. We haven't used the OR since I've been here and that's been almost two years."

We stepped inside a room that looked like a museum of medical artifacts. A metal surgical table, rusted and green with age, sat in the middle of the room surrounded by stained, wooden counter tops and cabinets covered with dust. Chipped tiles lined the walls and floor and a heavy surgical lamp, coated with grime, hung from the ceiling directly over the table's center.

"Take a look at this," Sally said. She nodded to a steel cart parked in a corner. "Do you know what this is?"

"Of course. It's an old anesthesia machine."

"There was a time this thing passed gas," Sally said. "But I'm told there haven't been any gas anesthetic agents here in over five years."

I inspected the machine for anything I could use. There were two tanks lying on their sides on a bottom shelf of the cart. One was marked halothane, the other nitrous oxide. Neither was connected to a regulator and both appeared empty.

"The only tank I know of that's ever been connected to the machine is the O2 tank."

Sally pointed to a third tank, larger than the two on the cart, which *was* connected to a regulator. Operated correctly, it could deliver oxygen.

"Try it," Sally said.

I turned a black knob connected to the tank's regulator and oxygen began to flow. I instantly heard a hissing sound.

"What's that noise?"

Sally held up two fluted tubes that connected the oxygen tank to a face mask.

"Leaks," she said.

I could see what she was talking about. Much of the oxygen flowing from the tank was leaking out through holes in the anesthesia tubing. Someone had tried to seal the holes with adhesive tape, but it wasn't working worth a damn.

"Count the patches," Sally said.

Twenty-two.

"We put in a requisition for new tubing six months ago but it never arrived. Finally, one day with nothing better to do, we taped each hole in an attempt to stop the leaks. We wasted our time."

I shook my head in disbelief. "What about deliveries?" I asked Sally.

"They have to go to Anchorage or Kotzebue. And to make matters worse, the airlines won't fly anyone within a month of their due date so all pregnant woman have to be away from their homes and families at least thirty days."

"That's outrageous," I said. "We're going to have to do something about that right away."

Sally then took me on a tour of the six inpatient rooms, the nurse's station, the so-called lab and X-ray, and then down a flight of rickety stairs to the cafeteria and radio room.

"You want to grab a cup of coffee?" Sally asked. "I have time since we have no inpatients. Your clinic patients start arriving about nine o'clock."

"You mean zero nine hundred hours," I said. "I'm an officer in a Uniformed Service now and gotta get used to all that kinda stuff."

Sally just grinned.

"I haven't had a cup of coffee since we landed in Nome on Saturday. I'd kill for one."

"Then you're my kinda guy," Sally said. She took me by the arm and led me into the cafeteria where I was hit with the aroma of fresh bread and a brewing pot.

Sally poured us both a cup and we took a seat. We chatted until 8:45 when I told her goodbye and headed up the stairs to face my first day of clinic.

CHAPTER 18

Twelve patients had arrived, yet clinic wouldn't open for another fifteen minutes. I knocked on the clinic door and stepped inside a small foyer.

"May I help you?" asked a middle-aged Eskimo woman dressed in a colorful top and white slacks.

"I'm Dr. Tom Sims, your new physician."

"Oh my God!" the woman turned and shouted. "He's here, everyone. He's here."

"My name is Esther," the woman said, turning back to me. "I'm your clinic assistant."

Two more people came in. One, an older white woman with fiery red hair and freckles, and the second, a young Eskimo girl.

"I'm Jamie," the redhead said. She pointed over her shoulder. "This is Maureen."

Both women shook my hand.

"I'm your X-ray and lab tech," Jamie said. "I'm also queen of the hospital so get used to it. Maureen here does all the paperwork for your clinic."

We all smiled and chatted a bit when Esther finally said, "I think we better get started. Everyone in town and all the villages know you're here. I bet we'll have over sixty people come in today."

"We have sixty people on the schedule?" I asked.

Esther looked confused.

It was Jamie who understood what I was getting at.

"Tom . . . er, may I call you Tom?" Jamie asked.

I nodded. *Of course.*

"People here don't really take to a schedule, so we don't use one. Clinic is just first come, first served. We usually run about forty-five to fifty when we have a doctor, and that doesn't include people who drop in from villages once the mail planes arrive."

"That's a hell of a lot of patients for one day. What's this about mail planes?"

"Local airlines make mail runs from Nome out to surrounding villages three times a week. They almost always come back to Nome with a few patients who want to see the doctor."

"Sometimes villagers just come in on their own," Jamie added. "Other times they're ones you've authorized during radio traffic."

"Radio traffic?"

"They really didn't give you much training in Anchorage, did they?" Jamie said, shaking her head.

I shrugged. "They told me how to survive mosquitos in a plane crash and how to let people choose eyeglasses. I never heard anything about radio traffic. I don't even know what that means."

"Bastards!" Jamie said. "PHS sends you guys out here to the bush with no idea what to expect. Let's get started seeing patients, and during lunch—we'll eat no matter how many people we have lined up—I'll show you the radio room and fill you in on what you've got to do."

Given two exam rooms and a small space where I could hand write clinical notes, Esther and I made it through twenty patients before Jamie busted into my work area and announced our lunch break.

"Cafeteria—now!" Jamie ordered.

I saluted, set down my pen, and followed her downstairs.

I grabbed a quick sandwich and a glass of real milk. Both were delicious. It was the first chow I'd had in three days, other than my daughter's baby food and a few packaged snacks, and I felt guilty for eating without sharing with Pat and Grama. Halfway through my sandwich, Jamie told me to gather up my eats and follow her.

At the far end of a darkened corridor, we came to a door with a hand-printed sign that read Radio Room. Inside, a stack of dusty electronic equipment hummed and crackled. Light in the room flickered as the electronics sucked energy from the town's power grid I had no doubt was frequently overloaded. Occasionally, a broken, unintelligible word or two came through a small speaker mounted on a table next to a microphone. It sounded more like static than actual human voices.

"This is where you'll hold radio traffic every morning," Jamie said. She pulled a clipboard off a nail and showed me a list of village names with letters and numbers written after each one.

"You are medically responsible for thirteen Eskimo villages within a 150-air-mile radius of Nome. It's your job to contact each of these villages seven days a week using this two-way radio and here's a list of the villages and the call letters you use to reach them."

Many villages on the list had odd names that looked very Eskimo to me: Shaktoolik, Unalakleet, Savoonga, Elim. Others had more English-sounding names: White Mountain, Teller, Gambell.

"The Public Health Service has trained one person in each village to act as a health aide. Each health aide has a radio in his or her home much like the one here. Seven days a week, villagers line up at the health aide's door and present symptoms. Then every morning, usually starting about seven o'clock, you are expected to radio each of these villages and talk with the health aide. You'll be given symptoms and that's how you are supposed to make a diagnosis and render treatment."

"You must be kidding!"

Jamie shook her head. "I wish I was."

"How much training have these aides had?" I asked.

"About as much as you had in your Arctic survival course."

Oh crap!

"Can they give me clinical findings, blood pressure, pulse, temp, physical exam findings?"

"Some have had more training than others. John, on Little Diomede, can listen to a chest and sort of describe what he hears. He can also take temps and describe draining ears in kids. Others are pretty well limited to talking on the radio and giving shots of penicillin."

"Wow," I said. I couldn't think of much more to say.

"There are lots of sore throats and draining ears in Eskimo kids," Jamie said. "The PHS wants you to prescribe ten days of daily penicillin shots for every kid who gets something like that."

I shook my head. "That's brutal."

"That's PHS medicine."

"Shit."

"Village health aides also have a very limited pharmacy in their homes. I'm told they have a little codeine, some ampicillin, lots of injectable penicillin, and probably some first aid supplies."

"What if I can't tell what's wrong with a patient over the radio?" I asked.

"Then you authorize them to come into Nome to see you. Hence my comment about the mail planes. If you think the problem can't wait for the next mail plane, you charter a flight to go out and pick them up."

I was almost speechless. "I've never seen or done anything like this before."

"Oh, it gets worse," Jamie said. "If you think a patient's condition is so critical they can't be transported by air . . . then *you* get to fly out to them."

"What in God's name could I do in an Eskimo village to help a patient so sick they couldn't be brought to the hospital?"

Jamie grinned. "Beats the hell out of me. That's why you earn the big bucks."

I paused a moment to gather my thoughts.

"So, how am I supposed to make these radio calls? Have you seen other doctors do it?"

Jamie nodded. She reached down and picked up the microphone.

"Watch this," she said. "This is KIC-736 Nome Hospital calling KMM-712 Gambell. Any copy?"

The radio hissed and grumbled. I heard nothing intelligible.

Jamie repeated her call.

Suddenly the radio burst to life.

"This is KMM-712 Gambell. I copy . . . Nome Hospital. Come back."

Jamie handed me the microphone. "Say something."

Jamie showed me a button on the microphone to push and I stammered. "Hello . . ." I looked down at the list on the clipboard. "Hello KMM-712 Gambell. This is Dr. Tom Sims. KIC . . . er something or other . . . at Nome hospital. I'm the new doctor in Nome. I'm just calling to say hello."

I looked sheepishly over at Jamie and shrugged. She grinned, teasing me for the familiarity with which I spoke, as if chatting on a phone.

"You don't need to repeat who you are or give the call letters once they've responded," Jamie said. "Just talk normal."

"Hello, Doctor," the village aide responded. "What did . . . say . . . me again?"

Shit, I couldn't understand a word she said. This was never going to work.

"Try again," Jamie said.

"Sorry, Gambell. I can't understand you. Please repeat."

More static and then the radio went dead.

Jamie took the microphone from me and spoke. "This is Nome Hospital, Gambell. We are doing a radio check. Thanks for responding. Nome Hospital out."

"Do I say 'over' and all that stuff you see in the movies?" I asked Jamie.

"You do if you want to stay out of jail. No kidding aside, this is high-level radio transmission and protocols are pretty strict."

Something more to learn. I should have taken notes.

"Everyone has trouble when they first begin," Jamie said. "You'll get used to it."

"I doubt it."

"No, you will. It's very dependent on weather. There's another radio at the nurse's station on the hospital ward. Because there is always someone on duty, that radio is on twenty-four hours a day in case of emergencies."

"So what happens at night if an emergency call comes in?"

"The nurse does her best to deal with it, but if she can't she sends someone out to get you."

Sends someone out? That's right. I forgot the BIA house doesn't have a telephone. I'm praying our permanent housing will.

"Twenty-four hours a day?"

"Seven days a week," Jamie answered with a smile.

I shook my head. I wasn't sure I was going to be able to take all this in.

There was a knock on the Radio Room door.

"Dr. Sims," Esther muttered. "I know you're very busy, but we have over thirty more patients lined up to see you. More will trickle in during late afternoon. Do you think you could get started now?

I looked at Jamie with a very weak smile.

"Welcome to Nome," Jamie said with a grin. "We're so glad you've come. It's like the town motto says . . . there's no place like Nome."

CHAPTER 19

Pat and Grama were fast becoming experts at running an Arctic household. They learned to conserve water, avoid the honey bucket man when he was doing *his* business, and make do with the simple supplies and household items they had on hand. They learned to order emergency provisions from Anchorage and have them sent by US mail. What supplies and food they needed quickly and couldn't wait to get by mail, they purchased sparingly at the NC for twice the already inflated prices charged in Anchorage.

Because fresh milk wasn't available, Pat discovered Milkman, a powdered-milk product not as good as regular milk, but better than the condensed canned stuff we first tried. Fresh eggs could be bought and sent from Anchorage by mail. We thought that was crazy, but it was the way most people got them. Surprisingly, they usually arrived about 90 percent intact.

Dr. Hayden mentioned that I'd be making an occasional trip to Anchorage on official PHS business, so Pat began keeping a list of items I should pick up at the commissary at Elmendorf Air Force Base just outside town. My list would consist of items we used most, like cheese, canned bacon, lunchmeats, and flour for making bread.

I held clinic Monday through Friday, saving Saturday and Sunday for time with the family. It was difficult being on call twenty-four/seven, and I never had more than a few hours free at a time without being called to the hospital for some sort of emergency.

My first three weeks passed quickly. Clinic pace never slowed down, but I found myself adjusting to its rigors. I started radio traffic promptly at 7:00 and was usually finished by 8:30. I started later on weekends. I adapted to the finicky moods and sounds of the radio as Jamie promised, and unless the weather was particularly bad, I soon had little trouble understanding what the village aides were trying to tell me.

Evaluating symptoms and rendering treatment over the radio also got easier as my experience grew. I treated sore throats and earaches with scores of penicillin shots, and cringed every time I gave that order. I became adept at distinguishing sprains from fractures, colds from pneumonia, simple cuts from deep lacerations, and all types of minor infectious diseases that could be treated with one of my two antibiotic choices—penicillin shots or ampicillin by mouth. Rashes were particularly hard to diagnose over the radio, and I'm ashamed to admit that I succumbed to the habit of prescribing topical cortisone for just about every one presented to me.

By the end of the third week I had delivered five babies—two from women who lived in Nome and three from mothers flown in from surrounding villages. I considered doing deliveries in Nome a major accomplishment and was lenient in allowing pregnant women to fly on mail planes closer to their due dates than ever before. I was lucky. None of my expectant mothers ever had a baby in flight.

I developed a strong friendship with Jamie (our queen of the hospital), Esther, Gracie, Maureen, Sally, and all the nurses who worked various shifts. I got to know many of the volunteer DJs who worked at KNOM radio and, as Sally predicted, I fell prey to the influence of Father Poole and recorded several "Health Spots" that were aired all around the Seward Peninsula.

I did my best to stay away from Mr. McCoy. He did his best to stay away from me.

It was 5:00 A.M. and I had just finished delivering a baby. I was tired, and since radio traffic wouldn't start for a couple of hours, I decided to grab a little shut-eye in one of the empty patient rooms instead of taking time to go back to the BIA house to get some rest.

We had no inpatients, but night nurse Susan Simpson still had to remain on duty until her shift ended at 7:00 A.M. Around 6:30, she knocked at my door and offered me a cup of coffee. She asked if I was up for a little company. I reached for the coffee and motioned her in.

"Have you been here long?" I asked.

"Long enough," Susan answered. "This is my second and last year."

"Tired of the cold?"

"I'm from Minnesota so it's not the cold. It's the darkness that gets to me."

"Yeah, so I've heard. I wonder how it'll affect me."

"Better than me, I hope," Susan said.

For days afterwards, I thought about my conversation with Susan and the comments she made about Arctic darkness. I'd read about Arctic winters and realized they were long and viciously cold. But I'd never given much thought to how *dark* they would be.

Nome was about 140 miles south of the Arctic Circle—that latitude at which the sun never sets in summer, but where it likewise never peeks above the horizon during winter. As far as I could tell that meant Nome would soon be plunged into absolute darkness for twenty-three out of every twenty-four hours of the day and I never could have imagined how disastrous that would be to my spirit.

CHAPTER 20

It was shaping up to be the busiest clinic day yet. I was concerned about how long people waited because we operated on a first come, first served basis. So, even though I'd been advised against it, I asked Maureen to set up an appointment schedule. I wanted to see for myself how it would work.

Maureen hit me with an evil eye the moment I stepped into clinic. Thus far, we had forty on the books for the day, with another fifteen to twenty expected to just walk in. She couldn't wait to tell me how she felt about it.

"People not going to like dis schedule idea," Maureen complained. "People not like change. Me and Esther not like change, either."

I could see Maureen's passion in her eyes and it made me realize I was a visitor to their Arctic world, a person from a different culture. The last thing I should try to do was change people's way of thinking over to mine. The only way I was going to successfully adapt to this new life was to adjust *my* attitude, *my* thinking, and *my* actions rather than the other way around.

"Scrap the idea and go back to how you are used to doing it," I told Maureen. "You obviously know more about what people want than I do. I respect that."

Maureen came over to me and offered an uncharacteristic hug. "You good doctor," she said with a warmth I'd not heard in her voice before. "You goin' to do very well here in Nome."

By midafternoon we'd gone through forty-five patients. Both exam rooms were filled with screaming kids and the waiting area was standing room only. I was about to examine the draining ears of a panic-stricken four-year-old girl when Esther stuck her head through the exam room door.

"Nurse Helen says come listen to radio message from village health aide in Elim. Somet'ing goin' on. Helen seem very nervous."

I'd worked with Helen enough to know she was not subject to panic. She would never draw me away from a hectic clinic unless it was absolutely necessary. I excused myself from the girl's mother and hurried to the nursing station. Helen was there, holding the microphone and anxiously tapping her foot. She handed me the mic before I sat down.

"This is KIC-736 Nome Hospital calling KLM-749 Elim. Go ahead Elim?"

After a moment of irritating static, the village aide came in loud and clear. "This is KLM-749, Elim, village health aide Martha Aluke. Come back."

"Roger, I copy you, Martha. This is Doc Sims. What do you have?"

"Hello, Doctor. I have twenty-year-old male, Jimmy Aput, with severe stomach pain and vomiting."

"I copy that, Martha. How long has Jimmy been sick?"

"Jimmy say got sick last night after dinner. Threw up three times during night. Said he too sick to come to my house this morning when I hold sick call."

I looked at my watch. 3:00 P.M. He'd been sick nearly twenty hours now.

"Does he have a fever?"

"Yes, I took. One-hundred degrees."

Good. She took his temp.

"Any blood in his vomit?"

"No, don't t'ink so anyway."

"Please ask him," I instructed.

Thirty seconds of silence passed.

"Jimmy say no blood, but pain get worse after he puke."

"Where is the pain located?"

"Jimmy point all over his stomach. Worse around belly button."

Periumbilical abdominal pain of several hours' duration, accompanied by low grade temp and vomiting. Could be anything.

Diagnosing abdominal pain is always a challenge, but doubly so when trying to do it over a radio. The usual workup entails taking a good medical history and performing a careful physical examination that includes blood work and X-rays. I was expected to do it with garbled words exchanged with an inexperienced, inadequately trained village health aide a hundred miles away

My mind raced through a differential diagnosis. Was it something potentially serious like an ulcer or appendicitis, or something relatively innocuous like stomach flu?

"Martha, take your hand and press around his belly button. Ask him if it hurts."

"OK," Martha said. "Please wait."

A few seconds passed and Martha answered: "It hurts everywhere I push, Doctor."

"Can you be more specific?"

"Don't t'ink so. Every time I touch Jimmy he cries out and pushes me away."

"Do you know where the appendix is?" I asked Martha. By this time, I could tell by her cracking voice she was starting to get worried.

"I t'ink so, Doctor."

"Try pressing around his appendix and see if that hurts."

Seconds passed again. "Jimmy says hurts dere and everywhere else in stomach. He says he feels like gonna puke again."

"Is he passing gas?" Often a bowel obstruction is associated with a quiet belly and no flatus.

"Passing gas?" Martha asked. "Do not understand passing gas."

"Farting?" I bellowed into the microphone. "Has the patient been farting?"

Helen punched me on the shoulder and gave me a thumbs-up for my choice of words. *It is an axiom of medical practice to speak in terms people understand. Helen understands the rule well.*

I could hear Martha timidly ask the patient, "Jimmy, Doctor wants to know if you been farting."

A short pause then: "Yes, Doctor. Jimmy farting."

So, it's probably not a bowel obstruction. Thank God for that. I consider asking Martha to perform a rectal exam on Jimmy, but decide it is probably something neither she nor Jimmy Aput would be comfortable with.

"Stand by a moment, Martha. I'll be right back on."

"Roger, Doctor."

I turned to Helen. "I can't tell what's going on without seeing him, so what do I do now?"

"Ask Maureen to call Munz Air and tell them you need a stretcher charter to Elim. She'll take care of everything."

I nodded.

"Martha, don't let Jimmy have anything to eat or drink. I'm sending out a charter that should be there in about . . ." I looked up at Helen who held up two fingers. ". . . two hours."

"Roger dat, Doctor," Martha said. Then she added, "Oops—gotta go now. Jimmy just puked all over kitchen table. This is KLM-749 Elim. Out."

The radio call to Elim took forty-five minutes. When I returned to clinic Esther was frustrated. "I try to send people home to come back another day," she said. "But everyone say they like you and want to wait."

I took the statement as a compliment and smiled. It felt good people were beginning to trust what I had to offer.

"You get busy now, and I see what I can do bout crowd waiting," Esther said. She turned and started out to the waiting area, then stopped and looked back at me. "Oh, almost forget. Mr. McCoy stop by and say for you to come see him before you go home today. He say very important."

It was just past 5:45 P.M. and we still had several patients waiting to be seen. I did my best to focus on the coughs, sore throats, painful backs, vaginal and penile discharges, but my mind kept slipping back to the abdominal pain I had coming in by plane. If it turned out to be a surgical case, I had no idea how I would go about handling it.

At 6:30, while scribbling my last prescription for the day, commotion rose up from the ambulance entrance near the hospital's rear doors. I handed the written script to the patient, thanked her for coming in, and headed down to see if it was Jimmy Aput. The hospital doors flew open and I was greeted by a huge man with the darkest skin, whitest teeth, and friendliest smile I had ever seen.

"You must be the new Dr. Sims," the gentleman said, extending a hand the size of a baseball mitt. I reached out and shook it, hoping he wouldn't fracture one of my metacarpals in the process.

"I'm Frank Brown, your local taxi driver and one of your two ambulance attendants." He took a little bow and I grinned.

I introduced myself, bowed in return, and expressed my pleasure at meeting him.

"I have your charter in the back of the ambulance," Frank said. "I'm not a doc, but he don't look so good."

Jimmy was pale. He still had a low-grade temp and writhed in pain every time I palpated his McBurney's point—that area in the right lower abdominal quadrant that is tender to touch in acute appendicitis. His bowel tones were normal, another sign he probably didn't have a bowel obstruction, and my rectal exam did not increase his pain.

"Please have Jamie do a complete blood count and urinalysis," I said to Helen. Those tests would help confirm or refute my suspicions about what was wrong with this young man.

Just as I completed giving my orders to Helen, the hospital doors flew open a second time, and in shuffled a middle-aged Eskimo woman slumped over at the waist. She was very pregnant, and the front of her skirt was so saturated with fluid that she left a watery trail as she lumbered down the hall.

"Husband out fishing," the woman cried out as I ran toward her. "Water broke ten minutes ago and baby coming now."

"How many babies have you had?" I asked the woman.

"Seven. Dis baby coming very soon." She leaned forward and grunted in a push.

"DON'T PUSH!" I begged the woman. "Let us get you into a bed."

I hollered for Helen to call Esther and rush the woman into the OR. If we didn't get her taken care of stat, she was going to drop her baby right on the hospital floor.

Before Esther appeared with a wheelchair, the hospital doors flew open again. There stood a young man, tall, thin and very blond, holding a blood-soaked towel over his right arm.

"What in the world happened to you?" I asked the young man.

"A truck motor fell on my arm. It's cut real bad, Doc. I think maybe it's broken."

"What's your name, son?"

"Jessie Clark."

"How old are you, Jessie?"

I slowly teased away one fold of the bloody towel as we spoke.

"Fifteen."

The wound began to ooze.

"Do your parents know you've been hurt?"

"One of my neighbors saw the accident and brought me up here. My dad works for Wien Airlines and the neighbor's gone to get him. My mom's in Anchorage."

Jessie flinched and inadvertently drew his arm away. "Sorry Doc!" he cried. "I don't want to be a baby, but it's really painful."

The boy impressed me. He was in serious pain, but cooperative and in control.

"I need to see what we're dealing with here so bear with me just long enough to get this towel off your arm."

"OK," he said. Slowly, I removed the remainder of the blood-soaked towel and inspected his arm.

A deep, jagged, four-inch laceration spread across the surface of Jessie's skin. The laceration oozed instead of pumped, suggesting that no major arteries were cut. Small bits of tissue, muscle fibers and, veins protruded from within the injury and I could see exposed tendons that controlled movement of his fingers and wrist. His forearm was unnaturally curved.

"It's a nasty cut," I told Jessie, "and, you're right. I'm pretty sure your arm is broken. First we need to get the cut cleaned up and then we'll take an X-ray."

"OK."

"I can have the nurse give you a shot for pain if you'd like."

Jessie nodded. "If it would help."

"It will. Once that's taken effect someone will start cleaning out the wound. Now I have a couple of emergencies ahead of you, and we're short-handed. So you rest here a while, and I'll get to you as soon as I can. Understand?"

Jessie nodded. "I do. Thank you, Doc."

"You look beside yourself, Tom," Jamie said. She handed me the results of Jimmy's lab work. "Stop and take a breath."

Hers was good advice. Here I was, stranded deep in the Arctic with three emergencies staring me in the face, each one demanding my immediate and undivided attention . . . and I was alone. I needed to relax and focus on what to do next.

I was just three weeks out of my internship and still felt wet behind the ears. Now, I was trapped in a situation where my skills and instincts were being put to the test.

It wasn't the first time I'd been faced with multiple emergencies to handle all at once. That happened at San Joaquin General just a few months before. My mind raced back, searching for what I learned that night that might be of help now.

SAN JOAQUIN GENERAL HOSPITAL
EARLY FALL, 1970

Stillness draped over the ER corridors like strands of a spider's web. A quiet night when the moon is full. Hospital lore held that such conditions were a setup for disaster.

I was moonlighting in the ER to earn extra money. The few patients we'd had over the last two hours had been nothing more than a couple of sore throats, one case of abdominal pain (that turned out to be gas that miraculously resolved with one giant explosion of flatus), and a child with asthma. I was grateful for such an easy night since I'd only been out of medical school for two months and hadn't yet acquired the professional skills to handle anything more complicated.

It was my third moonlighting ER shift since starting my internship, and the first shift I wasn't paired with a more experienced resident to bail me out if I got in over my head.

Phil Sartini, my closest friend and the other intern working with me that night, was beat. His face was drawn and pale as if gravity had worked overtime during the night. He was on his OB rotation and had spent the last twenty-four hours without a minute's sleep.

Phil was a bachelor from a well-off family in New York. His father was an obstetrician and his mother a lawyer. Phil really didn't need the extra money from ER moonlighting like many of us did. He picked up an occasional shift just to take the load off his fellow interns. He was that kind of guy.

"Why don't you go home and get some sleep?" I suggested. "It's a slow night."

"You sure?" Phil's expression showed that he was tempted. "Things can fall apart at any moment. There's a full moon out."

"Yeah. I'm sure. I'll have 'em call you if you're needed."

Phil reached out and gave me a quick hug. "Thanks, buddy."

I nodded. "It'll be our little secret."

Phil pulled off his scrub shirt, tossed it in a hamper, and walked out shirtless into the warm night air. A spark of envy shot through me as I watched him head out the door—good looking, fit, not a care in the world, no one depending on him. I had had that life not all that long ago. But then I remembered all of the good things in my life *now*: a loving wife, a daughter, a home that was kept in perfect order for me. I knew I was the lucky one. I smiled as I waved Phil off, but must admit, I sighed just a little as the automatic doors closed behind him.

I turned to Jan Peterson, the night nurse who was closing out paperwork on the child we'd treated earlier for wheezing. "I'm gonna grab a few winks in the call room. Wake me if anything comes in."

There are few places less desirable to sleep than an intern's call room. They are cold, dingy, lonely places; a far cry from the hot sex caves we see on our favorite TV doctor shows. Thus far in my career, I'd spent many nights in call rooms and had yet to get a good night's sleep in one. More than that, I had yet to see, hear, or participate in a single romantic interlude in a call room, for there was little in the ambiance of the place to spark even the slightest interest in romance.

It looked as if a little rest might be possible that night. But then, just after 2:00 A.M., a rock concert in nearby Stockton broke up, and hell discended upon San Joaquin General Hospital Emergency Room with a vengeance.

"It was crackling on the ER com radio that made me think something was about to happen," nurse Louise Peterson told me later. "That radio's usually completely silent unless something big is about to come down."

"This is Double A Transport," the ambulance driver said amid traffic noise and static. "Come in San Joaquin General. We've got a bad one here . . ."

"This is San Joaquin General, Double A. I've gotcha. What do you have?"

"Young woman suffering respiratory distress and smothered in some sort of goo. Damnedest thing I've ever seen."

"ETA?" Louise asked.

"Five to seven minutes."

Then: "Breaker! Breaker!" a different voice shouted over the radio. The frequency cleared. "This is Allied. We've got a young male, maybe a drug overdose. Not sure, no one's talking. He is currently having a seizure and he's covered with some sort of slime we can't identify. Vitals are unstable."

Within seconds, a third ambulance driver took over the airwaves and then a fourth. All described similar cases, all potentially fatal.

"Good God," Louise cried to the student nurse standing paralyzed next to her. "Run, get Dr. Sims. Hurry!"

"Dr. Sims, Dr. Sims . . . we need you in the ER right now. Ambulances are coming in. Lots of them."

I bolted from the call room carrying my shoes and ran to the emergency room. Automatic doors swished open the second I got there. I pulled on my shoes to rush out and meet the EMTs.

The first ambulance screeched in and slammed on its brakes. Before coming to a complete stop, its doors burst open and two EMTs leaped out. The first was holding an IV bag high above his head, struggling to keep it from tangling in the mechanism of the ambulance door. The other cradled a portable ECG machine in the crook of his left arm and a large black Ambu breathing bag in his right.

I rushed over to the gurney's side and looked down at the patient. What I saw horrified me.

The patient was a barefoot young Caucasian woman with a thin, wiry frame draped in a tie-dyed blouse and baggy jeans. Long, matted platinum hair lay plastered to her forehead and shoulders. She was covered in a strange mucoid slime and she smelled a concoction of vomit, stool, and urine. She was unconscious and in the midst of a grand mal seizure.

The EMT tried to keep an oxygen mask planted over her nose and mouth, but her flailing convulsions made it difficult. I could hear her gagging.

The most striking thing about her presentation wasn't the seizure. I'd seen plenty of those during my training and had become immune to the impact they had on my psyche. What got me most was the gunk that smothered her face.

What the hell was it? Had she collapsed into some sort of oil when the seizure began? I checked her hands. They were covered with the same murky ooze as her face, but not mixed with dirt as if she had fallen. I drew a dab of the slime onto my fingers, rolled it around to feel its texture. Sticky, thick like syrup. I recognized its smell as a mix of bodily secretions—snot, sweat, and saliva . . . all mixed together in a disgusting soup of human fluids. And she was drenched in it.

Her ears were draining a yellow, sticky substance. Earwax. Her hair was soaked in oily perspiration from the back of her neck.

Then I realized: the slime didn't come from something she had fallen in. She was actually manufacturing it herself. It was as if every pore in her body, every orifice, every gland capable of secreting fluids was doing exactly what it was biologically programmed to do. Make mucous.

One of the ambulance drivers attached an Ambu bag to the woman's oxygen mask and began squeezing. Bubbles rose at the mask edges indicating lack of adequate seal. He pressed the mask tighter to her face and squeezed again. More bubbles. Her chest didn't rise when he squeezed, a clear indication she wasn't being ventilated. Without oxygen, she would be brain dead in minutes.

"Doc," the EMT hollered to me. "I can't get air into her."

I grabbed the Ambu from the EMT and took control, as if I could do anything the highly experienced first responder could not. I squeezed the bag as hard as I could. My hand met resistance that indicated some sort of blockage was preventing air from getting into her lungs.

"Gimme a flashlight!" I shouted.

The EMT grabbed a light from his emergency kit and handed it to me. I slipped the oxygen mask from the woman's face and forced her mouth open.

"Give me something to prop her mouth open!" I shouted to everyone around me.

The student nurse handed me a towel. I wadded it up and stuffed it into the corner of woman's mouth. It did the trick. I could see inside.

The woman's mouth, throat, and nose were completely clogged by the same thick bloody phlegm that covered her everywhere else. If we didn't get it out, she'd be dead in minutes.

"Suction!" I hollered to nurse Louise who had come out to join me. "She's drowning in her own secretions."

Louise ran into the ER and returned with a suction machine. Connected to the properly sized tip, I could pass plastic tubing down into the young woman's trachea and, using this machine, remove blockage that was preventing her from getting air.

Louise flipped a switch and the machine roared into action.

"Now an oral airway," I shouted. Louise already had one ready to go.

Working a suction tip with my right hand, I reached with my left to take the airway from Louise. It slipped and dropped to the ground. The woman's seizure intensified.

"Goddammit," I cursed. "Louise, give her five of Valium IV. We gotta stop this seizure."

Louise went to work immediately.

"Five in," Louise said.

We waited a few seconds. Nothing.

"What the hell, five more."

Louise pushed another bolus of the clear yellow fluid into the woman's IV and within seconds the flailing of her body began to slow.

"Now, give me a fresh airway," I said. "And call Sartini. I'm gonna need some help here."

Louise bolted back into the ER and returned with a fresh airway. With the seizure slowed, I was able to tease the second airway over the woman's tongue and down into her throat. Now I had space to work. I eased the end of the suction tip down into her windpipe and worked it in and out like vacuuming a rug. It was like trying to suck Jell-O through a straw.

"I'm getting nothing. Crank the machine up!" I barked.

Louise checked connections on the machine and turned a dial. The machine shuddered as I worked the tip. The woman gagged and then her limbs began to thrash again in the seizure that wouldn't relent.

"Try to hold her down." I shouted out to the EMT standing next to me. "If I can't get this damn mucous out, we're gonna lose her. Louise, five more of Valium IV. Now."

"That'll be fifteen milligrams, Doc. A lot."

"Ain't gonna matter if she's dead."

Louise nodded and drew up another bolus of Valium. Just as she was beginning to inject the med into the patient's IV, we caught a break. The seizure slowed again.

"Hold off," I said. "She's calming down. Keep the Valium handy in case we need it later."

I felt we were making headway when unexpectedly, the suction machine quit. I withdrew the suction tip from the patient's throat and found its end plugged by a glob of slime. Excessive pressure and strain had caused the machine to cut. I checked the collection bottle. Empty. All my attempts to clear her airway had been pointless.

One of the EMTs had ripped open the woman's blouse in order to plaster two electrocardiogram electrodes onto her chest. She was in sinus tachycardia; her heart rate was rapid, but not fatal. If I could get some air past the mucous barrier and down into her lungs, there was a chance we could save her.

"Get me a tracheotomy tray. Quick!" I ordered.

Just then, an alarm from the heart monitor pierced the air. Her sinus tachycardia had deteriorated into ventricular fibrillation, a lethal arrhythmia.

I grabbed a set of paddles and smeared gel on the woman's chest.

"Clear!" I hollered and pressed a button.

ZAP!

The woman's body rose from the table, shook, then settled. I checked her monitor. Nothing. I told the EMT to increase the voltage and I shocked again. It worked. Her cardiac rhythm returned to a functional beat. Now all she needed was ventilation. We rushed her inside the ER so we could work more efficiently.

A second patient was then hauled into the ER and placed into a cubical. "We need ya, Doc!" the EMT grunted. "This guy's on his way out."

"Go ahead and check the other patient," Louise said to me. "We'll keep suctioning until Dr. Sartini arrives."

"OK. And start a Dopamine drip if her BP starts to fall."

"What about epinephrine?"

"Have an amp ready for intracardiac use," I said.

Louise nodded. I handed her the suction tip and told her to have Sartini check the woman the instant he got in.

I pulled on a fresh pair of gloves and stepped over to check the patient that was just brought in. It was a young male presenting with the same signs as the woman: obtunded, reeking of stool and urine, and drenched with unbelievable amounts of slimy bodily mucous. It looked as if his entire body was dissolving down into a sickening pool of grunge.

The first thing I did was assess the boy's ventilation. He was still dressed and so covered with sweat and slim I couldn't tell if his chest was moving or not. I pulled up his shirt so I could listen to his heart and lungs.

"Hand me a stethoscope," I said to the student nurse, who by this time looked as if she were ready to quit nursing school and join a convent. She reached in her pocket and timidly handed me her brand-new Littman nurse stethoscope, bright red with a small stuffed animal curled around one of its tubes.

I planted the stethoscope bell firmly on the boy's chest and closed my eyes. Nothing. I felt his neck for a carotid pulse. None. I buried my knuckles into his sternum to elicit a response to pain. There was none.

With hesitation, dreading what I was about to see, I raised one of the boy's eyelids and shined in a beam of light. His eyes were clouded over and glazed; his pupils were fixed and dilated.

All in all, twelve people were brought into the ER that night. They ranged in age from seventeen to thirty-five. Phil Sartini and I worked furiously, fueled by need and driven by instinct, to save people's lives. We lost four—three men and one woman. I prefer to think we saved eight.

The young woman I worked on first survived, thanks to the expert work of Louise Peterson and the EMTs. Phil successfully injected her heart with epinephrine while I performed a tracheotomy.

The young man was DOA—dead long before he arrived at our emergency room. I later learned from the police his name was Troy. He was the son of a local physician and a promising college athlete. He was nineteen years old.

The cause of the deadly incident was ingestion of LSD that had been cut heavily with strychnine. Strychnine was cheaper than raw LSD and mixing the two together was a wretched practice drug dealers employed to stretch the amount of "acid" used in each dose of the drug they made. If combined carefully, strychnine could give a quick buzz—the psychoactive effect people wanted from LSD. If used improperly, it could kill.

Neither Phil nor I had ever seen a case of strychnine poisoning, let alone a person drowning in their own bodily fluids. I had never performed a tracheotomy; Phil had never injected intracardiac epinephrine. We had no book learning, no lectures, no hands-on training to deal with the throng of issues we faced that night. Yet we saved lives because we trusted our *instincts*, based upon our training, to show us the proper path to follow.

French actress Isabelle Adjani said, "Today I trust my instinct, I trust myself." I think she had it right. Learning to trust my intuition and following my instincts was the lesson of that night at San Joaquin General. It would be a truth that would guide me through the trials and heartache I would face in Nome in the coming years, and through the challenges I would face during the remainder of my life.

CHAPTER 21

D oc, you better get in here!" Helen shouted from the OR. "The baby's crowning."

"On my way." Then to Esther: "Get some ice and pressure on the boy's arm and have Jamie grab an X-ray. I'll be taking care of the delivery."

"OK, Doc," Esther said. She held up fingers to remind her what to do.

I ran to the OR sink and began scrubbing my hands.

"Make it snappy, Doc!" Helen shouted. "I got no intentions of delivering this baby myself."

I cut the scrub short, blasted through the OR doors and threw on a pair of latex gloves. There was no time to don a surgical cap or sterile gown.

A mat of curly black hair was just presenting at the patient's vaginal opening. I steadied my hands directly below the mother's pelvis, and in one push the baby was delivered. There were no complaints of pain, no tears, no stitches needed. I suctioned the baby's nose and mouth with a bulb syringe and gave one gentle pat between the shoulder blades that elicited a strong, healthy cry.

"It's a beautiful baby girl," I said to the mother. I placed a plastic clamp on the umbilical cord, made a separating cut, then quickly examined the newborn to be certain she was fine. Satisfied all was well, I placed the baby into the mother's arms. She smiled but said nothing, then took the infant to her breast and began nursing.

The delivery took less than ten minutes. It was simple and beautiful the way nature intended.

"Put the mother and baby in a room and I'll check on them as soon as I see what's going on with the other patients," I said to Helen.

Helen nodded, and helped the mother move off the cold OR table onto a gurney.

"Jimmy's white count is elevated," Jamie said. "Fourteen thousand with a left shift. Urine is clear. You thinking appendicitis?"

"I am now."

I turned to Helen. "We need to operate, but we need more help. Who can we call in?"

"Sally has to work nights and we're going to have inpatients, so she needs to sleep. Connie just got off her shift."

"What about Gracie?" Esther spoke up.

I turned to Jamie who said, "She used to work the OR and she's good. Since we stopped using the operating room a long time ago, she's now just a hospital aide, but she could do it. Sally gave her some days off since we had no inpatients."

"Can we call her and have her come in?"

"No phones in Nome," Esther reminded me.

Just then Jimmy cried out in pain. "Can you give me something, Doc? I'm dying here."

"We've gotta get his appendix out before it ruptures," I said.

I looked at Helen. "Give Jimmy a hundred milligrams of Demerol and fifty of Phenergan. That should ease him up. And while you're at it, give seventy-five of Demerol with twenty-five of Phenergan to the boy with the injured arm." Then I turned to Esther. "What do you know about working OR and surgical instruments?"

"Enough to say I don't want anyt'ing to do with dem," Esther said. "Dat's Gracie's job."

"Then we've gotta get Gracie here."

"Send Frank to get her," Jamie suggested. "He knows where everyone lives. I think he's still here in the hospital cleaning up the ambulance."

"Great idea," I said. "Tell him to get her here fast."

I turned to Esther. "Can you clean up the OR from the delivery since we need it for the appendectomy?"

Esther nodded.

"His arm certain does look broken," Jamie said. "I'll get an X-ray as soon as I get a minute."

"OK." I suspected the kid had a Colles fracture—a common break in the forearm. If the X-ray showed one, it was going to require setting before casting or it would never heal properly. But Jessie also had that laceration that needed cleaning and suturing before I could ever begin tackling a fracture. The cut was very close to the bone, and if infection set in it could become very serious.

"Helen, how long has it been since you've scrubbed in on a surgical case?"

"Never." she said.

Shit. Shit.

"Never? Come on, didn't you get some OR experience in nursing school?"

"Oh, all right. Once or twice. But not since then and it almost made me faint. I didn't like it then and I wouldn't like it now. I'm a floor nurse and that's it."

"Esther, if I numb up this laceration with local anesthetic, can you clean it and apply a dressing?"

Esther shrugged. "Guess so."

"OK. Get me ten cc's of one percent lidocaine with epinephrine."

Esther nodded and shuffled off to get me the local anesthetic.

"Now," I turned to Jamie. "Please get an X-ray of the kid's arm once Esther has the wound cleaned and dressed. And please keep an eye on the boy while we're in surgery. If there's a fracture, I'll set and cast it as soon as we get out of the OR."

"You got it, boss," Jamie said, and left to wait until she could get Jessie Clark in for his films.

Waiting for Frank to bring in Gracie, I infiltrated Jessie's laceration with local anesthetic so Esther could go about cleaning it. The boy was cooperative in every way.

With Jessie's laceration under temporary control and the baby safely delivered, I could now think about what to do in preparation for my first surgery in the bush.

"Where the hell is Gracie?" I asked Esther. It had been over twenty minutes since Frank left to get her.

"Don't know, Doctor," Esther said. "Should take only five minutes to drive to Gracie's house. Maybe she not home."

"Let me know the minute she gets here. This appendectomy can't wait much longer."

Power digging through drawers and cabinets in the OR while we waited for Gracie was more productive than I expected. I found drapes, stacks of sterilized surgical instruments, a box loaded with suture material, IV fluids with needles and setups, and a host of surgical dressings. What I didn't find was medications.

"What do we have for anesthesia?" I asked Helen.

She scoffed. "We've never had a surgery in the time I've been here, so I have no idea. Far as I know there's only the lidocaine for sewing up cuts."

"Show me the pharmacy cabinet," I said.

Helen took me to a tall wooden chest I'd noticed sitting next to the nurse's station and unlocked its doors. We searched inside.

I counted several vials of Valium, two bottles of a potent antipsychotic medication called Thorazine, some containers of antibiotics, and an unopened package containing six bottles of ketamine.

I knew ketamine. It was an anesthetic agent we used at San Joaquin General, mostly for brief surgical procedures on kids. I ripped away the cellophane wrapper from around the anesthetic drug and checked the expiration date: February 1969. *Shit! Out of date by over two years. Too bad, it will have to do.*

Ketamine was great because it was easy to administer by intramuscular injection and it had few side effects. Though kids did fine with ketamine, older patients often suffered postoperative nightmares following its use. If ketamine was my only choice for Jimmy Aput, nightmares were a potential side effect I'd just have to accept.

"May I speak freely?" Helen asked.

"Always." I said. I stopped reading bottle labels and gave her my undivided attention.

"Surgical cases always get transferred to Anchorage. Shouldn't we just send Jimmy off and not try to operate on him here?"

Helen made a valid point. My gut said she wasn't right, but I understood her concern.

"This kid's appendix is hot as hell but I don't think it's ruptured yet," I explained. "He needs surgery right now. He can't wait until the next jet to Anchorage, and getting him there by charter tonight would be time-consuming and risky."

Helen considered what I said and nodded.

"What about anesthesia?" she asked.

"We'll use the ketamine. I'll combine it with some IV Valium and local."

Helen forced her shoulders to relax. "OK, then," she said. "You're the doctor."

I smiled and said to her, "Go change into surgical scrubs and begin washing your hands. You're about to become scrub nurse number one!"

"Oh, no! Please!"

"I'm sorry, Helen, but yes. We can't wait any longer for Gracie and you're the only one available to help. Remember what you just said: *I'm the doctor.*"

Helen huffed, then turned and headed off towards the nurses' dressing room. "Fuck," I heard her mutter as she stomped away. I turned my head so she wouldn't see me grin at her response.

Ten minutes later, Gracie came in. She was limping and had a scrape on her cheek.

"What happened to you?" I asked.

"House too small and I trip over dog. From now on, dog goin' to sleep outside."

"I know you've had OR experience, but I've already asked Helen to help me. Can you keep an eye on the new mother and baby while we're tied up?"

Gracie shrugged. "Sure." She nodded towards the hallway. "What's wrong with da kid lying on gurney?"

"He has a broken arm with a bad laceration. Keep an eye on him as well."

"You got three patients in all at once?" Gracie said. "Four counting da baby. Look like all hell break loose in Nome tonight."

Helen and I rolled Jimmy Aput into the operating room and had him move from the gurney to the operating table. The shot of Demerol mixed with Phenergan had helped his pain.

"Dis is cold on my ass," Jimmy said.

"You'll live," Helen growled. She really wasn't happy I was going to make her assist with the surgery. "Now scoot over so we can get you centered under the light."

Jimmy lifted his butt off the table and moved slightly left. He winced in pain as he moved.

Jimmy in place, I explained in detail everything we were about to do. Several times during my talk he drifted off so I knew the shot of pain medicine was doing its job.

I'd done several appendectomies during my internship, but always with a surgical resident at my side directing my actions should I start to make a wrong turn. There was always a skilled scrub nurse, ready to hand me the instrument I needed next (even if I wasn't sure what it was) and an anesthesiologist standing guard at the head of the table, monitoring the patient's heart and every breath.

Here it was just Helen and me with our blind ambition, hoping to do everything right to save this kid.

Jimmy was scrubbed and draped. I had started an IV and he was resting quietly. I calculated the correct dose of ketamine and pumped it into his left buttock.

"You ready?" I asked Helen.

She shrugged and said nothing. I didn't need words to know her real response.

I adjusted the overhead operating light directly over the place on Jimmy's abdomen where I planned to make my incision. I took a deep breath, relaxed my shoulders, and held out my hand for Helen to give me a scalpel. Then, just as I was about to make my cut into Jimmy's skin, we were plunged into total darkness.

CHAPTER 22

What the hell just happened?" I screeched.

The OR door popped open and Gracie flew in by flashlight. She knew I was going to be upset.

"Don't worry, Doc, dis happen all da time," Gracie said. "Jamie was taking X-ray of dat boy Jessie's arm and it caused too much power draw on da hospital circuit when you usin' da damn surgical light."

"Isn't there an emergency generator? This is a hospital for God's sake."

"Generator broke down two winters ago. No one fix yet."

Shit!

"We're trying to do a surgery here. What's it going to take to get us light?"

I knew my voice sounded like fingernails on a chalkboard. The power loss wasn't Gracie's fault but I was frustrated as hell. I fought the urge to step away from the table and throw surgical instruments against the wall.

"Jamie will call her husband Billy Koweluk. He a supervisor at da power company and good about gettin' power back on every time we lose it."

Every time we lose it. Son of a bitch, that doesn't sound good.

"How long will it take?" I asked Gracie.

"Last time bout two hours. Don't know about dis time."

Two hours! Screw that. If we waited that long, Jimmy's appendix could rupture. We had to come up with something quick.

Think. Improvise.

"Gracie, how many flashlights can you dig up?"

"I don't know, maybe three or four."

"Go do it. Once you've found as many as you can, get back in here with Esther, Frank, Jamie, anyone else who can shine a light and not faint at the sight of blood and guts."

To an outsider looking in, the scene would have been surreal. There we were, six people hunched over a body, four shining eerie lights as two dug though human innards like mad scientists working on a cadaver. I sliced and dissected skin and muscle then burrowed my way deep into Jimmy's abdominal cavity with my hands. Helen held retractors and watched for bleeders. I grabbed a wedge of bowel, drew it into the operative field and ran it through my fingers. There, I found my prize: Jimmy Aput's inflamed appendix just on the verge of blowing.

Suddenly, Jimmy moved! He groaned and lifted a leg off the table.

Oh my God, he's starting to wake up. Can't happen! I still have guts dangling out of his belly.

"Esther, shine a light on Jimmy's face. Quick!"

Jimmy's eyelids were fluttering, and his lips began to twitch. A deep frown had spread across his forehead. Damn it. They were sure signs the ketamine had run its course. If I didn't give him more in a few seconds he would wake up and rise off the table.

"Esther, you need to give one cc of ketamine in Jimmy's thigh and one-cc of Valium in his IV. Can you do that?"

A line of sweat trickled down Esther's cheek. I could imagine what her pulse must be doing. "Guess so," she whispered.

Jimmy moaned again and raised his leg again, higher this time. He tried to sit up and his abdomen jerked, nearly dumping his exposed colon out onto the floor. Helen swooned, and I hoped she wasn't going to faint. I heard Frank muttered something that wasn't quite clear.

With shaking hands, Esther drew up the anesthetic agents and was ready to go.

"Any place in his thigh?" she asked.

"Yes, Esther. Just give it. Now!"

Jimmy batted at me with his left arm and his body started to twist. We had seconds left before he'd be completely awake.

Esther plunged the needle deep into Jimmy's moving leg and administered the drug.

"Good. Now, draw up the Valium and shoot it into the IV port."

Again, Esther bravely followed my directions.

As if by magic, the grimace plastered across Jimmy's face began to relax. His eyelids stopped moving and he began to snore. Less than a minute later, he drifted down into full anesthesia, deep enough for Helen and me to continue our work.

I asked Esther to stay at Jimmy's side and check his blood pressure and pulse while Helen and I worked. With the additional doses of ketamine and Valium, we were able to complete the appendectomy without difficulty. I closed the abdominal incision with nylon sutures and applied a simple dressing that Martha could change back home in Elim.

"You did a great job taking care of Jimmy while we did the surgery," I told Esther. "I'll make an anesthesiologist out of you before you know it."

Esther looked up at me and smiled. "Don't count on it, mister."

"Well that was a first for me," Frank laughed. "I wasn't sure I was gonna make it when that fella started to wake up."

"Your help was very much appreciated," I said, and shook his hand for the second time that day. I imagined I would be seeing a lot of this fine man and I eagerly looked forward to it.

Helen was a basket case. "Don't ever ask me to do that again," she begged.

"Too much pressure?"

"Not enough training."

"But you did great. How about we spend a little time practicing together sometime and maybe we'll become a team."

"You'd take the time to do that for me?"

"Of course. Who wouldn't?"

Helen snickered. "You'd be surprised."

❖

"Sorry about the electricity thing," Jamie said when we came out of the operating room. "It never crossed my mind the X-ray tube could blow power in the whole damn place when you were doing surgery."

I nodded my understanding. "Did you get the film?"

Jamie held up one X-ray for me to examine and suggested I use the flashlight she held during surgery to look it over.

"I'd normally get two or three views. Lucky to get just this one."

The film told me all I needed to know. I was right. Jessie did have a broken radius. Esther had cleaned the wound, so I told Jamie I would go ahead and suture up the cut then take care of the fracture.

"That's going to be a bit of a problem," Jamie said.

"Why is that?" I asked.

"Jessie's dad got wind his son was injured and, while you were in surgery, came and picked him up. Esther had applied a dressing after she cleaned the wound and the father asked for a splint so I gave him one."

"Did you tell him we would take care of his boy right after we got out of the OR?"

Jamie frowned and shrugged but said nothing. I could tell by her expression there was more.

"Come on," I encouraged her. "What's up?"

Jamie paused.

"Come on. Tell me."

"The father said he didn't want some damn, inexperienced government doctor working on his kid. I had no choice but let him go."

Old feelings die hard. I wonder how long it will take me to overthrow the reputation of my predecessor.

"I guess there's nothing more to do then," I said. "Thanks for your help tonight. I hope your husband can get the power up before too long. We have inpatients now, and they need taking care of."

"My Billy's the best," Jamie said. "If anyone can get us going, it's him."

My feathers were ruffled by the actions of Jessie's father, but I couldn't let it haunt me. I'd never even met the man; I decided it was his problem, not mine. I checked on the new mother and baby by flashlight. Both were fine and sleeping peacefully. I did one last check on Jimmy and left post-op orders for Sally to follow during the night shift.

It was close to 10:30 P.M. I was tired and hungry and wanted nothing more than to go home. Despite what happened with Jessie's father, I was elated with what we had accomplished that busy, crazy night. We'd worked together as a team, handling bizarre situations and delivering with success we could be proud of.

By flashlight I found my way back to the clinic to pick up my jacket. Just as I was heading out the door, the note from Maureen, reminding me that McCoy wanted to see me at the end of clinic, caught my eye. With all that was happening, I had completely forgotten.

I grabbed my coat and headed out. I would talk with McCoy first thing Monday morning. If it was something really important, I figured he would look me up over the weekend.

CHAPTER 23

Pat was in bed but still awake when I got home. She made me a snack and over peanut butter and jelly I filled her in on the details of Jessie Clark's father and the power outage during surgery. She declared the teenager's dad an ass and told me losing power was something we'd better get used to. She marveled that I got through the night without going crazy.

By the time I got back to the hospital at 7:00 A.M. the next morning, power had been restored. Radio traffic was light, and I spent most of my time chatting with Martha in Elim about Jimmy.

I was home by 9:30 and had just stretched out on the sofa for a few winks when a middle-aged Eskimo man knocked at the front door.

"Doc Sims?" the man asked.

I nodded and welcomed him inside.

"My name Sam Nanouk. Word has it you won't have much food till barge arrives. Is dat right?"

I nodded. *"Word has it." In just three weeks we've already become the subject of local talk. I figure it's something we'll just have to get used to.*

"I have offer for you."

"Please, sit down."

Sam took a seat but kept his eyes glued to the floor. He spoke very softly.

"I need help setting salmon gill net out in da ocean. Son usually help me, but he in Anchorage learning to be policeman. You help me, I give you half of first take. Could be many salmon . . . could be none."

"I'd love to help you," I told Sam. "But I know nothing about setting a salmon net."

"Easy. I teach you all you need to know."

"When did you want to do this?"

Sam checked his Timex. "Salmon running off coast today. How bout now?"

Now? No time to get ready, although I'm not sure what "getting ready" really entails.

"Let me ask my wife," I said. I started towards the bedroom when Sam stopped me.

"White men need to ask wife if dey can go set salmon net?" Sam muttered. The chuckle in his voice was obvious. "I will never understand white man ways."

I shot him a grin and shrugged. Different men, different cultures. "Just let me run it by her and I'll be with you in a minute."

Pat, Chantelle, and Grama were stretched out on the double bed. Grama was reading. Pat was awake but curled on her side with Chantelle cradled next to her.

"Any contractions?" I asked.

Pat shook her head.

"I have something to ask you."

Grama pretended to keep reading but I caught her eyes peeking at us as she struggled to catch every word I said.

I explained Sam's offer. "We could use some food, and it would be fun for me," I said.

Pat began to pout but Grama stepped in.

"Tom's been working really hard, honey." She turned to me. "How long do you think you'll be gone?"

I shook my head. "Don't know. Never helped set a salmon net in the Bering Sea before."

"Oh just go ahead and do it," Pat grumbled. "I know you want to."

"You sure?"

Pat sighed then rose from the bed and took me into her arms. "I'm sorry I'm bitchy. I'm just really tired of being pregnant. Go have fun. And bring us home some food."

I kissed her hard and patted her on the rump. Then, with stocking cap on my head and jacket over my shoulders, I bolted with Sam out the front door.

"It's called an umiak," Sam said when I asked him about his odd-looking boat. "It's made of reindeer skin, dried many months then stretched over wood frame. Many Eskimo men have one. We use for fishing and hunting seals and walrus. Sometimes whales."

The boat resembled an artifact you'd see on display at the Smithsonian. It stretched about twenty feet long and spanned five feet wide at the mid-section. Two wooden benches straddled the interior and a small outboard motor was hitched onto the transom. A pile of nets, stacked high on the bow, shimmered in the afternoon sun as the boat rested on a small, two-wheel trailer attached to an old pickup truck.

I helped Sam back the umiak down to the water.

"Try not to get wet when you climb aboard," Sam said. "You get wet, you be cold whole time we work."

I nodded my understanding.

Sam was skilled at backing his trailer and releasing the boat. Once in the water, I held tight to a bowline while he pulled the truck and trailer from the water and parked along the sand.

"Now, draw boat close to shore so we can load gear," Sam said.

The boat was surprisingly lightweight and easily maneuvered. We loaded a couple of nylon bags and some fishing tackle from Sam's truck into the boat, then I climbed onboard so Sam could push us off the beach.

It seemed like risky business, motoring out into the open ocean in a boat made of scrap wood and animal skin. A musky odor, rank enough to irritate my eyes, wafted up as if the boat had been stored with fish guts rotting in its hull. I muttered a prayer that the boat didn't leak, and if it did (which I considered most likely), I prayed that we could be seen from shore and rescued before it sank.

"Where's the best place to drop the net?" I asked Sam.

He shrugged. "No one place better dan any other. I usually go out a mile or two where sea is deep. Dat's where we set net. We come back tomorrow and maybe have plenty of fish. You look worried. Maybe bout my umiak. I do dis many years like father and grandfather. Just sit back and enjoy ride."

One pull on the starter rope and the engine coughed to life. "She might look old," Sam said, nodding at the motor, "but I take good care of her and she reliable as hell. Just like my wife . . . who I never ask if I can go out and lay salmon net."

Sam skillfully piloted the boat and in less than an hour, he was satisfied with our position. I wasn't quite so sure. One glance over the horizon and back towards shore justified my concern. Dry land was nowhere to be seen.

"Dis is place we set our net," Sam said.

I wondered how he could tell with no compass or signs on the horizon to indicate our position. But Sam was certain and I figured it was just the Eskimo way.

Sam showed me how to feed the net over the side of the boat so it wouldn't tangle. Every few feet, he had me tie a buoy to the net's top header and lead weights to its bottom. The buoys and weights would keep the net properly positioned for snagging fish as they swam by.

"Do we anchor the net to the ocean floor?" I asked Sam.

Sam shook his head. "Sea current stable dis time of year and no storms comin' up. Net will be here tomorrow when we come back."

Who was I to argue? Sam and his ancestors had been doing this for generations. In less than two hours, our work was done and we headed back to shore.

The next day Sam knocked on our front door at twelve noon, sharp.

"You ready to go get net?" he asked.

I nodded.

"Wife let you go again today, two days inna row?"

"I'm a lucky man," I said with a smile.

"Den let's go. Today different. Today my bones tell me big storm comin'. Umiak strong boat, but not so good in storms."

Crap! I could have gone all day without hearing that.

We launched the umiak from the beach directly across from the BIA house. Chantelle was down for a nap, so Pat and Grama scurried out to watch us. A wind had come up, and the boat whipped about in the lapping waves. I held tight to the bowline as I had done the day before, but it wasn't as easy as then.

We climbed onboard without getting wet and I waved to my family as they shook their heads. I knew they thought we were crazy, heading out to sea with an Arctic front coming in. But I didn't mind. I wanted to impress my girls, to prove I could take care of them. It was Neanderthal testosterone all the way.

Heavy clouds, piling up against the western horizon, gave birth to high winds and choppy water. The chop grew into waves, then swells that sent surges of frigid, Arctic seawater over the edge of the umiak and onto our feet as we powered through them. The little motor groaned against the strain caused by the changing current.

We trudged without speaking through the rugged waves for over an hour. Finally, Sam spoke up.

"Seems like I tell small lie yesterday."

I turned to hear him better through the blowing wind.

"About what?" I asked.

"Dis is where we drop net yesterday, but it not here today."

"Could someone have taken it?"

Sam shook his head. "Everyone know dis is where Sam Nanouk drop net every year. No one ever bother other people's nets. Become outsider in community if dey did."

A wave slapped against the bow of the boat, drenching me. I shivered and pulled up the collar of my jacket.

"What then?"

"Sea swells bigger today den usual during salmon season. Wash net away."

"You're kidding!"

"Not make joke when can't find salmon net. You bring gloves?"

I frowned. "You didn't tell me to bring gloves."

Sam shrugged as if he didn't care. "Net can't be too far away. You keep eyes to right side of umiak; I watch left. You see somet'ing dat look like tangled buoys, you holler to me."

I kept my eyes glued to the horizon on the right side of the umiak as Sam directed. A clap of thunder filled the air; so close and so intense it caused the umiak to shudder. Then lightning fired across the sky and it started to pour. More waves splashed up, deepening the pool of water collecting at our feet until my shoes were completely soaked. After a few minutes, I could no longer feel my toes.

We searched for fifteen minutes and found nothing. Then thirty. Over the hum of the tiny outboard motor, I heard singing and turned to see Sam chanting a prayer. His expression was deep with concern, as if his petitions were divided between finding our treasure and keeping us safe.

A flash of white suddenly caught my eye at the peak of a swell. It vanished into the wave's trough in an instant, but I was almost certain what it was.

"Sam!" I shouted and pointed. "I think I see a buoy."

Sam raised a hand to shade his eyes.

"You sure?"

"Enough I think we should check it out."

"Den we go have look."

Sam revved the engine and headed where I pointed. We circled around through churning water until Sam finally spotted it, a mass of white tangled buoys that could only be the net we'd set the day before.

Sam steadied the boat as close to the tangled mass as he could and motioned for me to start hauling in the net. Then he hollered, "Wait!"

He reached inside a nylon bag and tossed me a pair of canvas gloves.

"For doctor who forget his gloves but can't get hands injured," he smiled. "Now you get busy and earn your fish while I keep dis umiak from sinkin' to bottom of da sea."

Forty-six flopping silver salmon slithered about our hull as we headed back to shore. According to Sam it was a great first catch. To me it was a terrifying experience but I had taken a risk and it was worth it. I'd made a friend in the Eskimo community that would help build my relationship with the people I served, and I'd brought home food for my family. It made me feel we could actually make it in this crazy place, even live off the sea if need be, until our barge arrived.

CHAPTER 24

On Monday morning, I finished radio traffic early enough to grab a cup of coffee before patients started pouring into the clinic. I figured I'd better haul over to McCoy's office now and get our meeting over with before he pitched a fit and ruined my entire day.

"Sit down," McCoy said. No good morning or inquiring about my family. Not even any courteous questions about how my first few weeks in Nome had been.

"I have two issues to discuss with you. Neither is pleasant."

I took a seat across from his desk and got comfortable. I considered asking him to be quick; I had work to do and needed to get to it.

"Issue number one." His tone made me feel like a school kid sent to the principal's office. "I had a Mr. James Clark come by my home Sunday morning to file a complaint against you."

"A complaint?"

McCoy nodded. "I don't particularly appreciate getting complaints about your work as I am not your employer. Nor do I appreciate disgruntled patients coming to my home, especially on weekends."

"What was the complaint?" I asked.

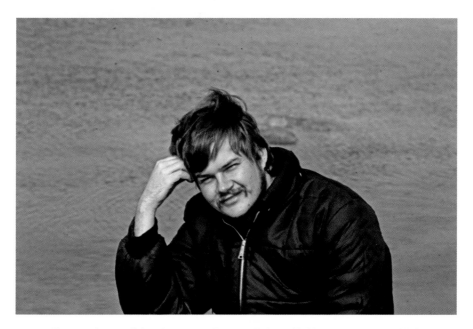

ABOVE: I'm wondering if there's any way I can pull this off. I have a two-year old daughter, a pregnant wife, and I'm expected to perform feats of medicine and surgery I have no idea how to accomplish. Coming here might be the biggest mistake I have ever made in my life. BELOW: Pat, nine months pregnant and moving to the Arctic. What were we thinking?

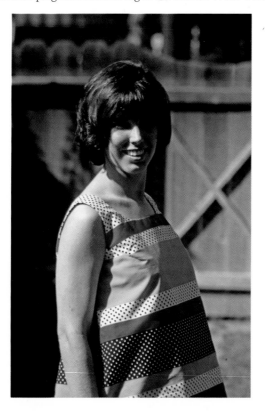

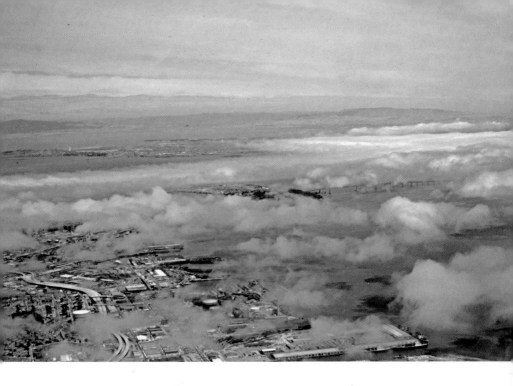

ABOVE: Our first aerial view of Anchorage that gives us a peek into our new life. BELOW: Our first view of the treeless barren landscape of Nome. It was far from what we expected the Arctic to be like.

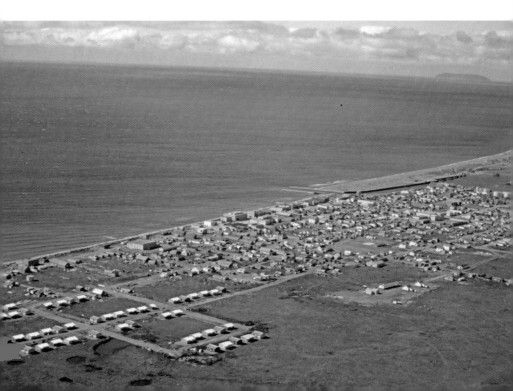

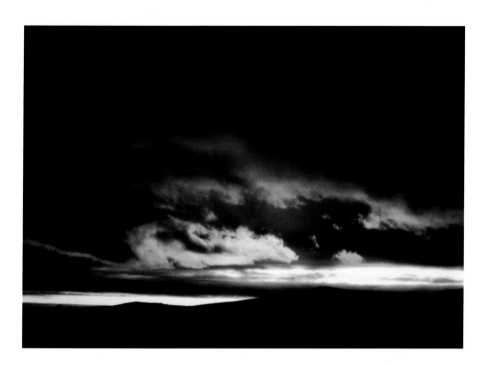

ABOVE: A summer Arctic sunset over the hills outside of Nome. The midnight sky is as dark as it gets in Nome during the peak of summer. BELOW: One of the nicer homes in Teller, Alaska, about seventy road miles north of Nome. It was the only Eskimo village we could reach by car during summer. Driving to Teller from Nome has an estimated driving time of nearly three hours to cover the seventy miles.

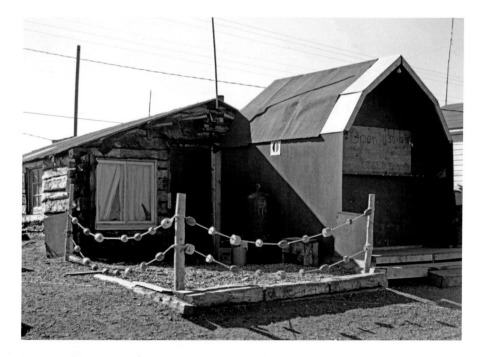

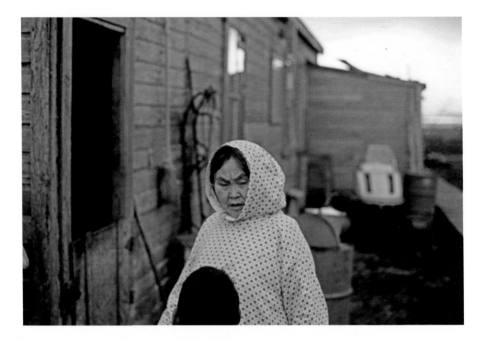

ABOVE: Eskimo grandmother outside her village home dressed in a typical warm weather dress known as a "summer parky." BELOW: Alaska King Salmon like they grow them up north.

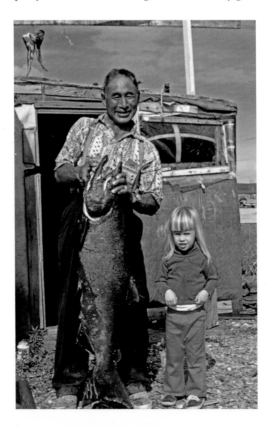

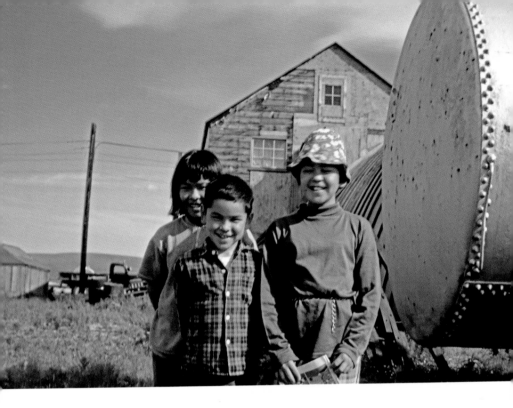

ABOVE: Smiling faces of beautiful neighborhood kids in Nome. These youngsters were Chantelle and Adam's first Alaska playmates. BELOW: A Cessna U205C Super Skywagon aircraft owned and operated by Munz Northern Airlines of Nome, Alaska. I flew in this plane so often I thought of it as my "second car." Otis Hammonds and Sparky O'Neil were my usual pilots.

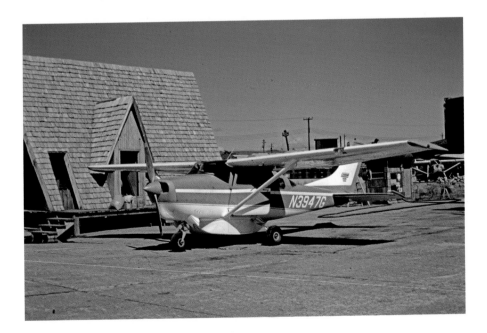

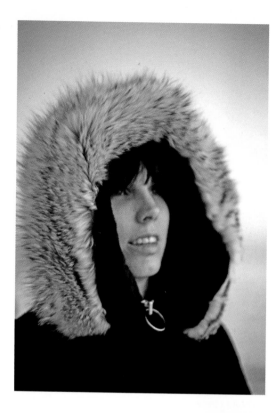

The face of our first Arctic winter arrived in style and beauty. My beautiful wife, Pat, in her mouton parky.

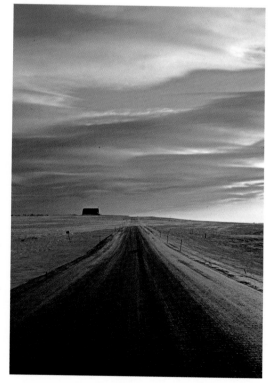

The one lowly paved road in town, heading out to the Roadhouse Restaurant twenty-two miles from Nome. I was traveling this road in winter when I had my snowmachine accident that injured my six-month-old son. The restaurant is still in business, now called the Safety Roadhouse Restaurant.

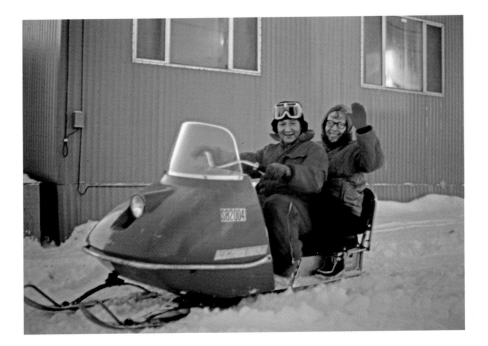

ABOVE: Beloved friends Billy and Jamie Koweluk, surrogate grandparents to our kids. Billy was head of Nome's power company and Jamie was our undisputed "Queen of the Hospital." BELOW: Tieuk, our Alaskan Husky. Born on the rocky shore of the Bering Sea, Tieuk was a genuine Alaskan sled dog, bred and raised in the Arctic.

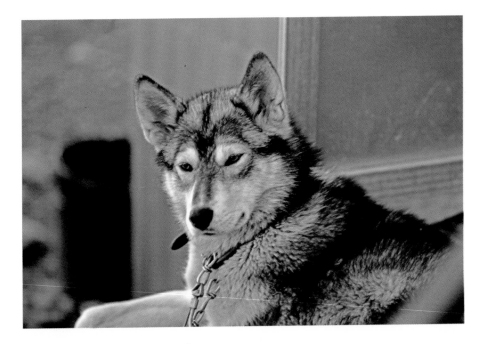

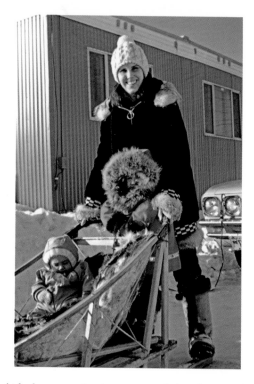

ABOVE: Pat with the kids demonstrating how we traveled with me pulling our dogsled using the Arctic Cat snowmachine. Pat is wearing her mukluks and mouton parky, Chantelle is in a slip-on parky with wolf ruff, and Adam is sitting on a reindeer skin sleeping bag. BELOW: Eskimo boats called *UMIAKS* made of reindeer skins stretched across a wooden frame. They are lined up for winter storage on the shoreline of the frozen Bering Sea.

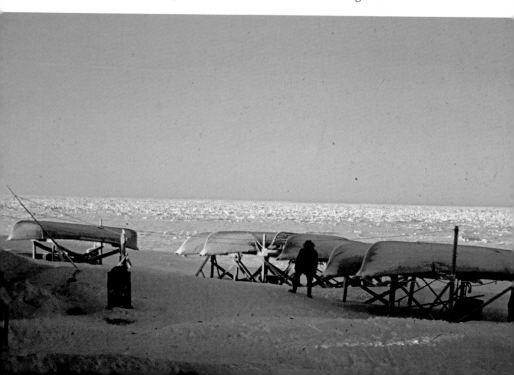

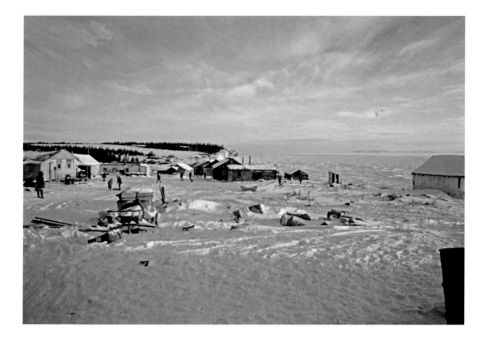

ABOVE: The Eskimo village of Elim—typical of where I went during winter for clinic visits—and one of my favorite villages because the people were so wonderful. BELOW: We load up on Jon Aluke's showmachine and sled then head into the Elim hills to find a Christmas bush.

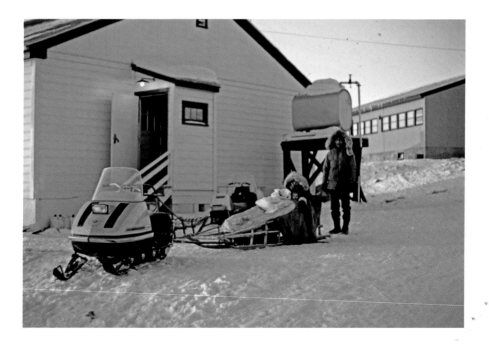

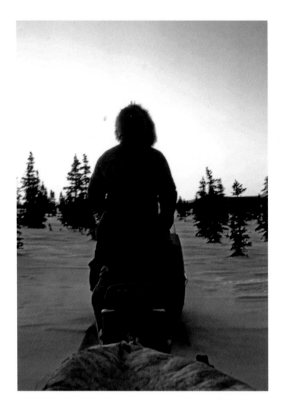

Jon drove. I sat on the sled with Pat and the kids holding on for dear life.

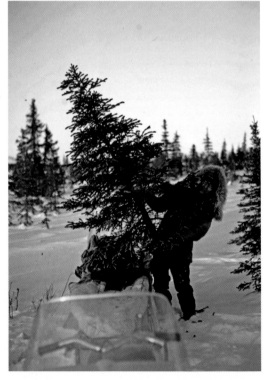

Success! And not bad considering what we had to choose from. You'll never believe how we got it home to Nome.

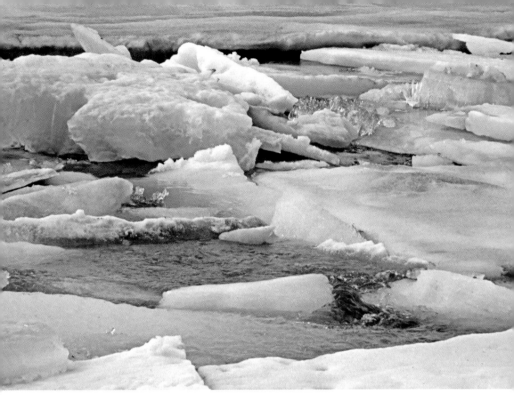

ABOVE: "Break up" of the Bering Sea is a natural phenomenon not to be missed. BELOW: Ice floes from break up provide hunting grounds for Arctic spotted seals.

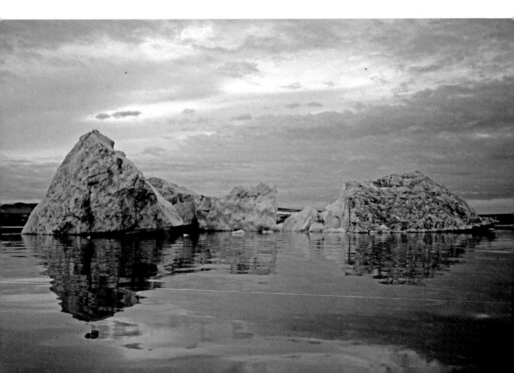

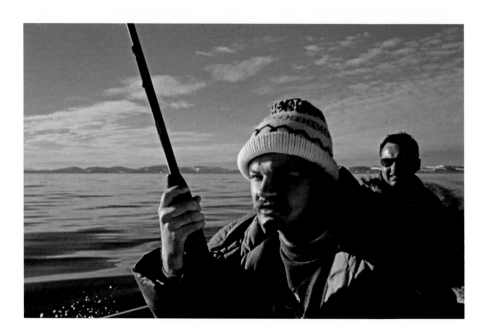

ABOVE: Floating among the ice floes with my buddy, Ed Greenberg, hunting for spotted seals. I wanted the pelts for mukluks. What happened next was a surpise. BELOW: Racks for drying Salmon, built on the shoreline to preserve the Fall's catch.

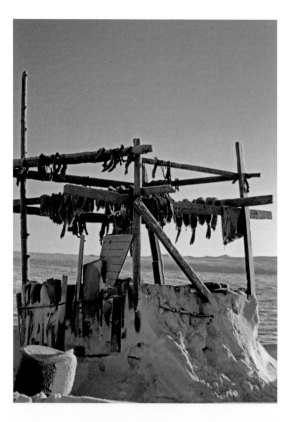

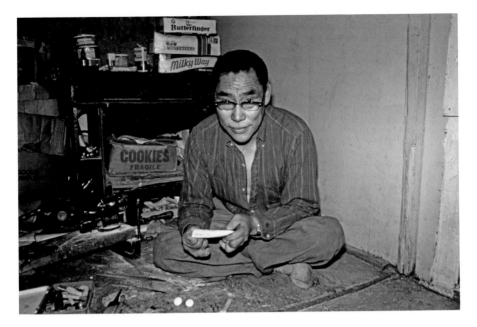

ABOVE: Daniel Iyakitan—a world famous ivory carver inside his home in Gambell, on St. Lawrence Island. Daniel's arthritis was so severe, he did much of his work using his feet. When I visited Daniel at his home, he taught me to carve a small whale of soapstone I proudly display in my Oregon home. Daniel passed away on March 5, 2008, years after I had the honor of meeting him. BELOW: The Native Store in Savoonga on St. Lawrence Island. Home of the sweetest people I have ever known. During one of my visits to St. Lawrence and its two villages—Gambell and Savoonga—I had the thrill of visiting Jacques Cousteau's magical boat The Calypso and meeting Philippe when the crew was on the island filming a TV special about walruses.

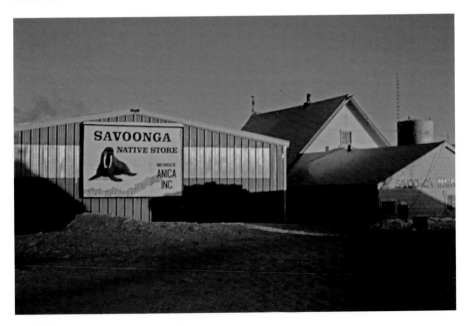

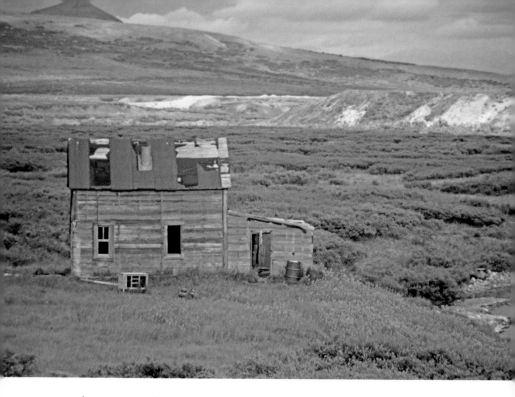

ABOVE: A summer seaside home located several miles outside of Nome. I never knew who lived there. Maybe it was Piccolo Pete after he abandoned his shack by the morgue! BELOW: On June 10, 1972 Pat and I decided to celebrate our fifth wedding anniversary camping on banks of the Sinuk River, about twenty-five miles over a gravel road from Nome. One hour after setting up our tent, we were plagued with a swarm of mosquitos the size of dragonflies and we had no choice but head home for safety. As I recall, we had frozen wieners and Pork and Beans for our anniversary dinner. It was the first and the last tent camping trip we ever did in the Arctic.

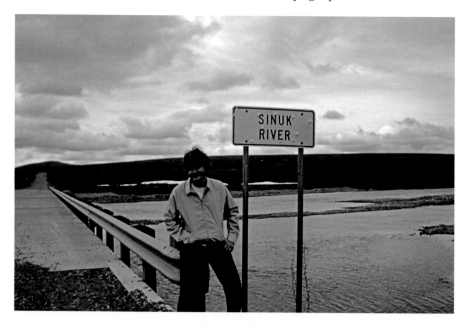

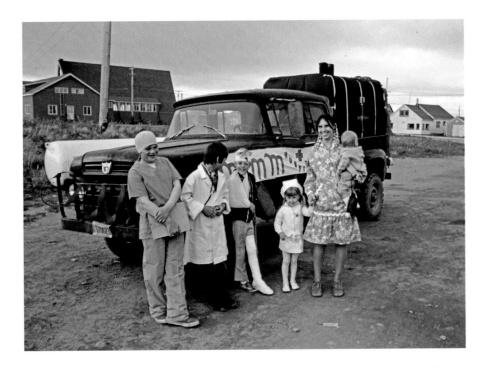

ABOVE: A Fourth of July parade celebration, Nome, Alaska style. Pat with our kids, our visiting nephew, Kevin, and two neighborhood kids. I drove the borrowed truck with an MMM Hospital banner plastered to the sides. Our "float" was a big hit but later we were verbally attacked by a local woman for becoming too much a part of the Nome community. BELOW: Our Husky, Tieuk, standing guard at the sounds of the breaking up ocean.

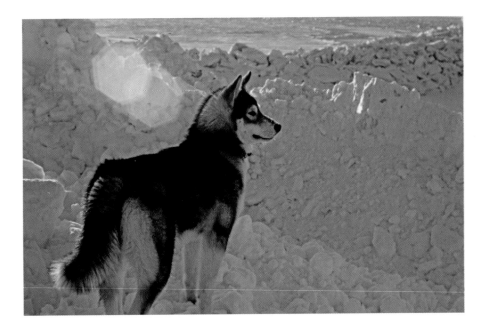

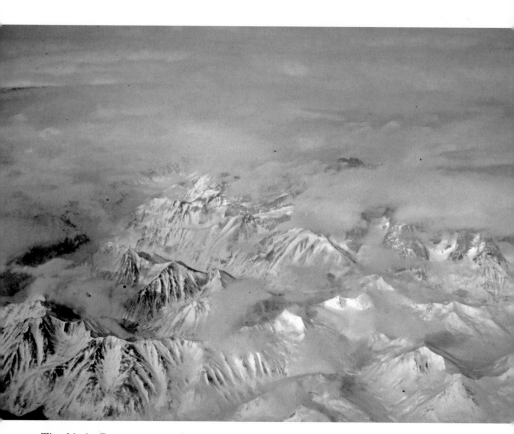

The Alaska Range as we made our final flight from Nome to a new home in Anchorage. It seemed strange to once again see mountains and trees. Living back in the city was going to take some adjustment.

"Mr. Clark claimed he brought his son in to see you Friday night with a serious injury and you brushed his son aside to deal with other, less serious patients." McCoy paused a beat. "*Eskimo* patients, Mr. Clark stressed. He says you left his son suffering terrible pain and serious bleeding."

"That's crazy."

"I have no reason to dispute what Mr. Clark says."

"Well you should," I said. "It's bogus."

I was taken back by McCoy's accusation, but more so by the fact he seemed ready to believe Jessie's father without first hearing my rebuttal on the matter.

I explained the situation in detail to McCoy: how I had three emergencies all come in at once and how I prioritized each according to their immediate medical need.

"I specifically told the boy I had two emergencies to take care of first and that I would get to him as quickly as I could. He understood perfectly."

McCoy didn't seem impressed.

"Mr. Clark has an entirely different take on the evening," McCoy said.

"How so?"

"He said you decided to take care of the Eskimo patients first, claiming it was your duty and what you were paid to do. He said you told the boy if he gave you some money, you would move him to the front of the line."

I stood and considered bolting from the room. "That's horseshit!" I growled. "I said nothing of the sort. And as a matter of fact, I never even *saw* Jessie's father or spoke with him personally. He and his son were gone by the time I got out of surgery."

"So, you did not give preferential treatment to the Eskimos?"

"Of course not! Anyone there Friday night can vouch for that."

"Well, let me make something perfectly clear, Dr. Sims. This hospital was built as a mission to service the needs of all people—white and Eskimo. Even the occasional black person or Mexican who might come along. But we can only do it with money we receive from private pay patients. We get very little from the PHS for work we do for Eskimos."

"Work *I* do!" I corrected him.

"Work *we* do," he persisted. "And if we don't make our paying patients happy . . . well, we just won't be able to stay in business."

I was so furious I had no intentions of discussing the matter further. I had taken good care of all the patients that night—including Jessie Clark—and felt no need to defend anything I did.

"You may want to sit back down," McCoy said. "You will have some interest in the other subject I have to discuss."

There was a tap on the administrator's door and Regina, McCoy's secretary, stepped in. She handed her boss a folder and he dismissed her with a wave of his hand. He opened the folder and removed a couple of pages.

"I received a message from PHS housing in Anchorage on Friday. I don't know why they keep bothering me with your housing needs as it is not my problem." He slurped his coffee, allowing a thin waterfall to dribble down his chin. He wiped it with the back of his hand.

"Perhaps it's because I don't have a telephone or receive any mail yet," I suggested sarcastically.

"Humph," McCoy muttered, then went on. "Whichever it is, it's your problem and not mine. At any rate, they wanted me to inform you that the BIA teachers will be arriving on Wednesday and you must vacate the BIA house by tomorrow noon."

"Tomorrow! That's nuts. I can't do it. I have a full work schedule this entire week and my wife could deliver our baby any moment."

"Once again, not my problem." McCoy said with arrogant, undignified satisfaction.

"Did PHS suggest where we are supposed to live?"

McCoy tossed two pages from the folder over to me. "I'm very much opposed to this arrangement, but apparently my hands are tied."

The papers revealed an agreement that had been reached, not with McCoy himself, but between a controlling board of the hospital and the PHS Department of Housing in Anchorage. According to the paperwork, PHS would be renting the currently empty doctor's house, owned by the hospital, for us and there was nothing Mr. McCoy could do about it. We were authorized to move in immediately.

"That's fantastic news," I blurted out. "I only wish there wasn't such a rush."

"Don't get too excited until you read the small print," McCoy said. "This is only temporary. Once I am able to obtain a private physician you will need to move out on the spot. Where you'll go is none of my concern and if you think . . ."

I couldn't keep from interrupting him. "I won't hold my breath for that to happen."

"For what to happen?"

"Finding a doctor to come work for you," I said.

"Well you better just . . . "

As far as I was concerned, the meeting was over. I got up and left his office, trying not in the least to hold back the grin I felt spreading across my face.

I scurried to the clinic and gathered Esther, Maureen, and Jamie for a quick meeting. Helen came over to see what was happening.

"We have to cancel clinic tomorrow," I told everyone.

Esther gasped, "We can't."

"We have no choice. McCoy is kicking us out of the BIA house so we have to move. The good news is we get to move into the doctor's house."

Esther shook her head. "Dat Mr. McCoy have somet'ing against you and da PHS."

Maureen agreed. So did Jamie and Gracie.

"To be fair, it's not all his fault. The teachers will be arriving in a couple of days and the BIA house *is* for them."

"Yeah," Jamie said. "But that doctor's house has been vacant for years. McCoy could easily have let you move in there the day you arrived if he'd wanted. He just didn't."

"Dat's true," Gracie added.

Helen shook her head. "All that animosity has gotten so much worse since that doctor came down from Kotzebue and got into all that trouble."

"But I'm not Jack," I said. "I wonder when everyone is going to stop comparing me to him."

Jamie stepped over and laid her hands on my shoulders. "We all know you're not him. You've been proving that every day. It's the town that needs to catch up."

Esther and Maureen nodded.

"Don't worry, it'll happen," Helen said. "Just keep the faith."

❖

That night I told Pat we'd needed to start early the next morning packing up all our things for the move. I tried to soften the blow by telling her how much nicer the "doctor's house" was going to be. I didn't get very far. She was too tired and too pregnant to see anything positive about all the work we'd be saddled with for the next few hours.

The bedroom clock read 7:15. I'd spent a restless night, still pissed about Jessie Clark's father and concerned about the clinic I'd have to make up because of cancelling in order to move. When I finally did get to sleep it was like anesthesia and 7:15 was the latest I'd stayed in bed since arriving in Nome.

I climbed out of bed to the warble of voices coming from the front room. I figured something was up at the hospital and Frank had come to fetch me. I cursed under my breath as I threw on a pair of jeans and T-shirt and went to check.

I was ready to spit nails when I saw Pat at the front door speaking to Billy Koweluk, Jamie's husband.

"What's going on?" I muttered. Foremost on my mind was a cup of coffee.

"Have a look outside," Pat said. She had the biggest smile on her face I'd seen in days.

I opened the door, and to my amazement saw a line of vehicles: cars, trucks, Frank's taxi, the Nome ambulance, a motorcycle, and even a pickup truck with Alaska Airlines logos embossed on its doors. Standing next to each vehicle was a person; some I'd met and others I didn't recognize. At the front of the line stood Jamie and Billy.

"What in the world is going on?" I asked Jamie.

"Word has it you could use a little help moving today," Jamie said with arms outstretched to exchange a hug.

It was the most welcoming sight I could have imagined. Pat rushed outside and hugged Jamie and Billy and waved everyone inside. "I'll make us all some coffee," she shouted.

Gracie then spoke up. "And I have cake!"

Everyone crowded into the house, met Grama and praised Chantelle for what a beautiful little girl she was. Helen and her boyfriend Don poured coffee into paper cups that Don had brought from the radio station, as Gracie, Esther, and Maureen served cake on paper towels. Even Regina, Mr. McCoy's secretary, was there. I could tell she felt uncomfortable until I gave her a hug and said I was glad she could make it. Father Poole from KNOM was there to bless the food and help.

"Now, you and Mrs. Sims sit down and tell us what to do," Billy Koweluk said quietly. "You do so much for all of us. In return, we all want to show our appreciation by doing somet'ing for you."

It took less than two hours for all our possessions to be packed up and moved to the doctor's house. Pat and I didn't lift a finger. Pat instructed everyone where various items went in the new residence, and by the time a lunch of salmon sandwiches rolled around, we were settled and ready to begin life in our new Arctic home.

CHAPTER 25

A neighbor loaned us his mini-sized Honda motorcycle. Pat was skeptical when I tried to convince her that using the bike for a rugged little jaunt over the tundra was just what she needed to jumpstart her labor. She was now a week overdue and it was starting to get her down. I'd always been told a bumpy car ride had worked for my mother when I was born. I was convinced the same would work for my wife.

I wasn't sure the two of us could fit on the tiny seat of the bike. But after some creative maneuvering, we did it. Once we got going, crossing the tundra was like motoring over a field of foam rubber covered by marshmallows.

The underpowered little bike spit and groaned under our combined weights as we bounced over ruts and inched up molehills. But we trudged ahead, spinning wheels and throwing bits of dried grass and lichen in our path.

Pat squealed when we grabbed tiny amounts of air then landed in a soft puff of sound. We crept over rocks, sped up over plateaus, and spun and twisted when I felt it safe and secure to do so. The ride was jarring and bumpy, exactly the labor-inducing course I was hoping for.

We tipped a couple of times, but never went over. We had fun, laughed, and enjoyed the freedom we shared. Sadly, Pat reported, there was no positive report from her obstinate uterus.

Five nights later I *felt* the tap on my shoulder more than I heard the whisper in my ear. I thought it a dream, rolled over and closed my eyes.

"Tom, wake up. I'm having strong contractions. I think I'm in labor."

I sat up and switched on the bedside lamp.

"They started about an hour ago and they're every two minutes now."

"I should check you," I said.

Pat nodded.

I rushed into the bathroom to grab a sterile glove and Betadine. Pat prepared herself with a towel beneath her bottom and knees raised.

"Oh my God!" I exclaimed. "You're about eight to nine centimeters dilated. Why didn't you wake me sooner?"

"I wasn't sure it was actually labor. I thought maybe . . ."

"Never mind. We need to get to the hospital right now or we're gonna have this baby on the bed!"

Reality of what was about to happen hit me like a sledgehammer. We were about to have a baby, isolated and alone in the bush of Alaska. *Even though I am the physician, I am the father as well . . . and there is no one for me to call!*

My head flooded with images of all that could go wrong. What if Pat hemorrhaged? Was a blood transfusion doable in Nome? Did the town even have a blood bank? What if the baby failed to rotate and was therefore vaginally undeliverable? Or what if the baby was breech and suffered oxygen deprivation or brain damage at birth? Would Pat ever forgive me? Worst of all, what if a life-threatening emergency happened, and the only solution was an immediate caesarean section? Could I detach myself enough from the situation to perform a section on my own wife?

It was Pat's idea to have the baby in Nome and to have me perform the delivery. She felt we had a duty to the community to prove I was a competent physician, and having our baby in town was a fine way to accomplish that. It seemed like a great idea at the time. But now, with delivery staring me straight in the face, it seemed like the stupidest dumbass decision we had ever made.

I took a deep breath, knowing I needed to control my anxiety. Panic was not going to help. I needed to completely relax and get the job done. And thankfully, I knew exactly what I needed to make that happen.

I rushed to the closet and grabbed our emergency delivery kit. I tore through the bag until I found what I wanted: the small brown Rx bottle that contained only one pill: Valium 5 mg.

I knew if I gave it too much analytic thought, I'd bail on the idea. So, without waiting another second, I rushed to the bathroom, drew a tall glass of water and I tossed the tiny pill into my mouth.

Pharmacologic help should be on the way in less than fifteen minutes.

"Hurry," Pat hollered. "I feel like I need to push."

"Oh my God, don't push. I'll be right there." Then a new, wild concern hit me.

I've never taken a tranquilizer in my entire life. What will it do to me? My thoughts raced to my mother, how her speech slurred and her gait waivered when she was under the influence of her pills. What if the pill does the same to me? What if the Valium sedates me to the point I can't manage Pat's delivery or I actually pass out and leave her without any help at all? Goddammit anyway! Why did I take that motherfucking pill?

There was only one thing to do! I stuck my finger down my throat like a bulimic teenage girl, and with a few horrible retches, brought the tiny pill up into my mouth. Though covered with bits of slime and stomach acid, the Valium hadn't yet dissolved so the drug hadn't started to course through my veins.

"Tom, hurry! I think the baby's about to come."

I don't know what instinct drove me next except love for my wife and concern for her wellbeing. But Pat needed to be calm and in control too. So I bit the regurgitated pill in half, swallowed one portion myself, and handed the second half to her.

"Take this," I said.

"What is it?"

"Please just do it!"

With complete trust, Pat put the pill between her lips and swallowed.

"Now," I said, kissing her firmly on the lips. "Let's get this show on the road."

If Pat's water broke the baby would be born in less than minute. *Isn't that the way it always happens? We've waited all this time for nothing and now we have a mad rush.*

I boosted Pat up into the Jeep and we drove the two blocks over bumps and potholes to the hospital. I begged her to breathe through the contractions and try not to push. She told me to go screw myself.

We pulled up to the hospital and made our way in. Nurse Connie Addison was on duty, and the moment she saw the look on Pat's face, she knew exactly what was up.

"Oh, God," Connie moaned. "Why does it have to be on my shift?"

"Never mind that," I said. "She's pretty close. Get her into the OR while I scrub up."

Connie took Pat by the arm and started to put her on a gurney.

"I don't think there's time for that. I really feel a need to push."

"DOC!" Connie hollered. "She wants to push."

"Tell her not to. I'll scrub and be right in. Do you know how to do a pelvic check?" I hollered to Connie.

"Oh, God no!" Connie barked back. "I hate OB and I hate my life."

"Just get her up into stirrups. But keep an eye on her and be ready to catch if necessary."

I heard Connie sigh but let it pass.

I pulled off my T-shirt and threw on a scrub top. I rushed to the scrub sink and turned on the tap.

I pumped a dollop of Betadine soap into my hands and began scrubbing. I used a brush to clean under my nails and debride dead skin from my arms.

"Hurry, Doc!" Connie cried out from the OR. "You don't want me delivering your kid."

I heard Pat moan.

I was so fired with adrenaline I didn't think the half Valium had any effect. But clearly it did, for as I stood at the sink scrubbing, awareness of time became suspended and my senses dulled. I was mesmerized by the warm, running water as it gently massaged my hands and forearms.

My breathing slowed and I closed my eyes. I scrubbed and scrubbed and scrubbed—illogically thinking if I continued washing, engulfed in the deep caress of water coursing over my limbs, I could avoid the reality waiting for me in the next room. A minute went by, two, three.

"GET YOUR ASS IN HERE!" Pat screeched from the delivery area. "This baby is gonna hit the floor if you're not in here to catch it."

Pat's voice, and a shake of my head, quickened my attention. I rinsed my hands and rushed into the delivery room. Connie handed me a sterile towel and a fresh pair of latex gloves.

Pat gave one push and there it was; the blond capped occiput of my baby's head.

"Easy, honey," I whispered. Connie turned her head away, kindly avoiding intrusion into the intimate moment Pat and I were about to share. "I see the head. Careful. I'm going to try and do the delivery without an episiotomy."

Pat could not have been better. She panted to resist the urge to push until I asked for one more gentle squeeze. Now the head was delivered, and the baby's shoulder was presenting beneath her pubic bone. I gently placed my index and third fingers round the baby's neck and pulled towards the floor. The shoulder easily delivered just as it should. Less than a second later, the baby began to rotate and the other shoulder came into view. I grasped the second shoulder, slid my hands forward and carefully deliver the torso and legs.

The baby was face down as it should be. I rotated and saw with great emotion we had a son.

I clamped the umbilical cord, cut the connection to the placenta, and placed our baby boy into Pat's arms. The afterbirth delivered immediately. There was minimal blood loss, no distress, and no surgical incisions.

We beamed with tears of joy and relief. I saw Connie wipe her eyes when she handed Pat a small towel to clean the baby's face.

Pat placed our newborn son to her breast and he immediately began to suckle.

After a few moments Connie asked if Pat was ready to be taken back to a room. She offered to get a gurney.

"I'd rather walk," Pat said.

I grinned looked at my wife with the greatest sense of pride.

Pat held the baby in her arms, and together we walked from the OR to a hospital inpatient room. Connie asked if we needed anything, and when we said no, she thoughtfully left us alone to relish our private moments undisturbed.

We named our son Adam Cory. We slept together in the single bed for two hours, then Pat wanted to go home. No one, especially me, dared argue with her.

We wrapped Adam in paper towels because the hospital had no diapers. Pat covered him with a patient gown and tucked him into her jacket for the ride home.

"Coming?" she asked as she headed toward the ambulance entrance.

I nodded and grabbed my coat.

We were back home at the doctor's house before anyone even knew we'd even left.

CHAPTER 26

I f I were asked to blueprint the perfect mother-in-law, I would only need profile Pat's mom and my job would be done. Grama was everything a man could hope for in a mother-in-law: kind, thoughtful, nonintrusive, loving. I had adored her since that moment we met in the elevator at UCLA.

Grama had put her Santa Monica life on hold in order to help us with our move and new baby. Never once did she complain of things being left undone in California. But she had a life outside of ours and it was time to get back to it. Grama asked me to make arrangements.

I selected a Sunday flight. That would give us one last Saturday together; a day I prayed would be quiet so I wouldn't be called away.

The day began early. Before any of us woke up, Grama had brewed a pot of coffee and had a fresh loaf of sourdough bread in the oven. We breakfasted on cold cereal and powdered milk, then, at Grama's request, I drove her downtown to the NC where we purchased cooking oil, butter, a bag of potatoes, a quart of real milk, and a chicken she would fry for dinner. Grama paid, saying no matter what it cost, she wasn't about to feed us another meal of salmon "cooked any way she could think of."

Late that afternoon we savored the warm sizzling smells of chicken crisping up in the skillet, and later the comforting taste of potatoes, mashed with butter and fresh whole milk. We relished the change in menu and enjoyed light conversation around the table. After eating we sat together quietly in the living room, the only noise a faint bubbling of the aquarium pump and KNOM playing softly in the background. We tried to read, but written words couldn't hold our attention.

We were pensive, pondering over the next day and what it would be like to have Grama gone. But Grama would have none of that. She lightened the mood by saying how boring life was going to be back in Santa Monica and her comment spawned joyful reminiscing about our last fourteen weeks together.

It took less than twenty minutes to load Grama's things into the Jeep and drive to the airport. We sat quietly inside the old wooden terminal building, Pat trying to read and Grama toying with the kids. Eventually, the flight was announced and it was time to say our goodbyes.

I went first.

"There's nothing I can say that comes close to expressing how wonderful it's been to have you here, Grama," I said. I gave her one last hug and wiped a tear from my cheek.

She also struggled to hold back her tears. "I wouldn't have traded this experience for anything in the world."

Grama kissed Chantelle and Adam and gently caressed their heads. "You take care of your mommy, now," she said to Chantelle, who seemed to understand something significant was about to take place. Chantelle began to whimper.

A simple goodbye, mixed with tears and a hug were all Pat could muster. Grama understood. It was enough.

Then Grama grabbed her carry-on with purse attached and, with one final wave, walked out the door. She was the last person to board the flight.

We drove back to the doctor's house in silence, afraid the simplest words would open a floodgate of tears. Even Adam was quiet as the sways and rolls of the huge vehicle gently rocked him to sleep.

It was on that ride home it actually hit me. *We are here, in the wild bush of the Alaskan Arctic, all alone. Did I do the right thing hauling my wife and family to the end of the world? Should I have let the draft take me and leave my wife and family safe and comfortable? Was I selfishly thinking only of myself and my own well-being when I brought us here?*

I don't know the answers yet, but I know I'm about to find out. The time has come to either survive or succumb.

CHAPTER 27

There are two seasons in the Arctic: winter and summer. Winter is predominant. When summer *does* arrive, it hangs around just long enough to titillate the senses and then overnight, it gives way to an isolated land of darkness, ice and snow.

Since no houses had become available for us to rent, the PHS decided to ship us a manufactured home. It was what people called a mobile home or a very large trailer. We assumed it would be on the same barge carrying our supply of food and car but weren't sure. We'd been on edge since hearing a barge headed for Nome from Seattle had suffered a fierce storm and much of its cargo had been lost at sea. We prayed our barge was not involved.

October had come and still there was no sign of our shipment. Winter freeze was threatening, evidenced by chunks of ice that floated down ocean currents from the pole and piles of ice along the Nome shoreline. Should winter set in and the ocean freeze completely over, we would never receive our ride, our food, or a place to live.

On a Friday afternoon toward the end of the month I was called to the hospital phone. Shirley Harper, the PHS housing agent Anchorage, was on the line.

After a few exchanges of pleasantries through static and crackles, Shirley told me to expect a barge in Nome the next morning carrying our new manufactured home. I was instructed to check for damage and report my findings to her. After my inspection, if the home arrived in satisfactory condition I was to sign a bill of lading, retain a copy for my records, and mail a carbon copy back to Anchorage. At that point, a team would be dispatched from Seattle to assemble the home on a vacant lot near downtown procured by the PHS. The job would take a week, and once completed, we'd be free to move in.

Shirley made no mention of our personal shipment or car, but since Housing wasn't involved with the shipping of personal goods, I wasn't concerned. I'd just have to inspect our own personal items once they were offloaded from the barge to be certain they arrived intact as well.

I began radio calls at 7:00 the next morning and by 9:30 had discharged all three patients I had in the hospital. Receiving our home, our personal goods and our car was going to be exciting, and I was eager to leave the hospital and start the day.

Connie was working day shift and I told her I would be at the harbor receiving my shipment if she needed me. She promised to send Frank to fetch me should there be any problems.

I Jeeped back to the doctor's house and found Pat and the kids dressed, fed, and ready to head out to the Nome jetty.

"No rush," I said. "Sunrise won't be until 10:30."

We stood along the retaining wall of the city harbor and scanned the horizon. Wind was brisk and temp near freezing. The sky was free of clouds, so rays from the brief Arctic sun warmed the chill on our faces.

Shortly after 11:00 A.M., we spotted a shape on the horizon. Through binoculars I could see it was a barge, loaded high and wide with stacks of huge box containers and large plastic-wrapped forms we guessed might be vehicles. We couldn't tell if a yellow Pontiac station wagon was included with the load. At the leading edge of the barge rested a giant rectangular object that could only be a manufactured home.

The barge crept along, leaving a trail of white foam in its path. As it got closer, it made a slow turn toward the Nome jetty, then stopped.

It took about thirty minutes for a tugboat to connect to the barge and settle it in at the dock using ropes the size of my arms. When the barge was stabilized, a large crane stirred awake and, with the help of several longshoremen, the methodical task of unloading began.

My heart sank when the first thing taken off the barge was a badly damaged manufactured home. A sticker plastered on a broken window identified the trailer as belonging to a local construction company. Unfortunately for them, the storm had taken its toll on their proposed building.

Next, one half of a large manufactured home was unloaded, and twenty minutes later a second half. I spotted a sticker plastered to the front of a large picture window that read "Property of the US Government" and knew our home had arrived.

We waited another hour as many box containers were unloaded and stacked on the harbor dock. I inspected each one and found my name plastered on the last one that came down.

Next came the plastic-wrapped vehicles. Third to last was a pale-yellow Pontiac station wagon with a familiar California license plate clearly visible through a fold of plastic that had ripped loose in the wind. Our car.

"Sign here," the harbor attendant instructed me. He handed me a clipboard with several pieces of paper attached. "Last page, bottom line."

I flipped through pages of legal jargon and read a few highlights. It was only the last page that gave me any concern.

The phrase read "Accepted in satisfactory condition . . ." and I pledged my honor and responsibility for accepting the manufactured home with an invoice price tag of $250,000!

The following week, a team of three workers arrived and went to work putting together our new trailer. They told me the home was specifically designed and constructed for the Arctic and contained insulation, electrical and plumbing components, even exterior walls and a roof built to withstand the prolonged subzero temps of Arctic winters. The house was the most expensive manufactured home ever built—and that didn't include the exorbitant cost of barging it up to Nome. It would turn out to be the nicest home in town.

CHAPTER 28

We were losing our daylight and I did not like it.

How dearly I loved those midsummer days when nature gifted us with twenty-three hours of sunshine out of every twenty-four. I loved the feel and taste of the late-night air as it caressed my face, the way its fragrance tickled my nostrils when I drew it in. Now daylight was shortening by six minutes every day and its loss affected my mood. Weariness descend over me like a cloak, a vail that bore witness to the fact our Arctic world would soon be engulfed in near-total night.

My mood should have been better. We had moved into the beautiful double-wide trailer and were settled at last. We had our provisions—clothing, food, and all the items we needed for the baby. We had the car, although little need for it considering how busy I was and how few roads there were to travel.

Clinic had taken on a life of its own. Since Adam's birth, people began trusting my skills and dedication to the job. Word was spreading, even to the doubtful non-Eskimo residents of Nome who had now started coming to clinic for care instead of heading to the airport.

Being accepted was gratifying at first. But the stroke to my ego was short-lived as the heavy, unending workload had begun to be a burden. As the only physician for three thousand people in Nome, plus another three thousand in the surrounding thirteen Eskimo villages, I had no life outside of being a doctor.

We still had no phone, and late one cold November Saturday morning Nurse Sally had Frank deliver a message to the trailer. A villager in Elim had sustained a deep arm laceration the health aide felt required immediate attention. A mail plane wasn't scheduled into Elim until the following Tuesday, so I had two choices. I could charter a plane to fly out to Elim, retrieve the patient and transport him back to Nome. Or I could charter a plane for myself, fly the ninety-five miles out to the village, repair the laceration there, and fly back the same day. Option two required only one chartered flight, plus I saw it as an opportunity to take care of a problem that had arisen at home that desperately needed my attention.

"Throw a couple of things in a day bag, grab the kids and your knitting, and let's all fly out to Elim," I said to Pat. "I need to charter out there today and the plane will hold all of us."

"What's going on in Elim?"

I explained about the man with the arm laceration but said nothing about the *real* reason I wanted her to join me.

"I could use a little change of scenery," Pat said. That was all I needed to hear.

"And grab a bedsheet," I said. "We may need one."

"Why?"

"Just grab one. I'll explain later, but we need to hurry. Otis has a Cessna waiting for us on the tarmac."

Otis Hammonds was the best bush pilot in the Arctic. Whenever we needed to fly locally, he was our number-one choice. If Otis said flying was safe, I was raring to go. If he said it wasn't, it was a completely different story.

Nome was on the verge of another big storm, yet Otis made the takeoff from Nome and landing in Elim smooth and easy. Upon landing we were met by an Eskimo man dressed in a fur parky and sealskin mukluks. He looked about forty, with a muscular build, burnt-butter skin, and coal black hair. He was riding a Ski-Doo snowmachine that he had connected to a beautiful hand-carved Eskimo dogsled. As he approached, he flipped back the hood of his parky, smiled, and extended a hand.

"I'm Jon Aluke," the man said, "husband to Martha, our village health aide. She ask me to come pick you up."

I pulled off a goose-down mitten and extended my hand. We shook vigorously. "Tom Sims," I said. "Doctor from Nome."

"I know who you are," Jon said. "Hear you plenty on radio calls when you talking to Martha. She t'ink very highly of you."

"I think very highly of Martha, too," I said, "and I look forward to meeting her in person. She is an excellent health aide and Elim is lucky to have her."

I introduced Jon to Pat and the kids. He complimented me on my girls, how beautiful they both were and what a handsome son I had. Then he said he'd like to take me to see Eddie Kikulo, the man with the injured arm. He motioned for us to climb onboard his dogsled.

"I'll wait here in the plane until you finished," Otis said. "Get back as soon as you can so the storm doesn't ground us."

"Will do," I said, and turned my attention to Jon's sled for our quick trip down to the village.

I took to the sled first and Jon motioned for me to scoot all the way back to lean against the musher's handrail. Pat sat next, between my legs. Jon picked up Chantelle and handed her to Pat who had gathered up a place for her in folds of her coat between her knees.

"Slip new baby inside parky," Jon advised Pat. "Den zipper back up so both you and he will stay warm for short trip to town."

Pat did as Jon instructed and nodded she was ready.

"Everyone OK?" Jon asked.

I checked Pat and the kids and shot Jon a thumbs-up. He fired up the snow machine with one pull of the starter rope and we headed down the hill toward his and Martha's home.

Martha Aluke was right about the severity of the injury. Eddie had been working on a snow machine engine and the wooden frame supporting it had collapsed. The engine crushed much of his right arm when it fell.

Eddie was lying face up on a mat of reindeer skins that Martha had draped over her kitchen table. A bloody towel encircled his right arm and he was moaning. A young Eskimo woman, who I assumed to be his wife, was wiping sweat from his forehead with a dishcloth.

I slipped on a pair of latex gloves and slowly unwrapped the towel. Eddie moaned, but held perfectly still so I could do what I needed to do. Once I could clearly see his arm, I was taken aback by the seriousness of his injury. The forearm looked like it had exploded from within because of a deep, jagged laceration that ran from his elbow to his wrist. I saw no shattered bone sticking through the wound and whispered a prayer of thanks for that.

Engine oil, clotted blood, dirt, and grime filled the cut, so I needed to clean the wound and remove foreign matter before I could start repairing it. My exploring fingers confirmed the injury was all muscular, with no bones, tendons, nerves, or major blood vessels involved.

During my training, such a severe injury would have been referred to plastic surgery. The patient would have been taken to the operating room where, under general anesthesia, the wound would have been cleansed, surgically debrided, and finally repaired. But here, in the kitchen of a remote Eskimo village during Arctic winter, such luxury was not going to happen. The repair of the wound was just up to me. I would have to improvise.

I had stocked my go-bag with everything needed to create a makeshift operating room in Martha Aluke's kitchen. I even had sterile surgical gowns and disposable drapes to create a sterile field.

Martha had a generator; I was relieved I wouldn't have to rely on flashlights or kerosene lanterns should the coming storm kill the community's juice. For this procedure to be successful, everything would need to fall into perfect place.

I required a surgical assistant to help with the operation—someone who wouldn't faint at the sight of blood and was skilled in surgical procedures and sterile technique. Someone like a zoologist would fit the bill. I looked at Pat and smiled.

Pat shrugged and handed our children over to Anna, Eddie's wife. She was more than happy to look after them. Adam began to fuss, but the moment Anna took him out of his mother's sight, he settled down.

Chantelle was well behaved and curious about the inside of the Eskimo home. Pat and I tied surgical masks over our faces, then scrubbed and gowned so we could get to work.

Raw nerves, left exposed in the wound, rendered it impossible to clean and irrigate the wound adequately for repair. We needed anesthesia.

Putting Eddie to sleep, even with ketamine, was too risky in a village aide's kitchen. Our only option was using more local anesthetic than I was accustomed to. I drew up ten cc's of the numbing agent lidocaine, diluted it with an equal amount of normal saline and, using the smallest needle I could find, infiltrated the skin and deep tissues thoroughly. Eddie winced in pain as the needle pierced his skin, but the sting of the medication quickly dissipated, replaced by the medication's numbing effect. I worried about side effects from the volume of local anesthetic it took, but Eddie tolerated the high dose without complication and did his best to hold still as we proceeded with our work.

Once the wound was cleaned and debrided, I gently opposed the deep torn muscle layers and sewed them together with wide looping stitches. I knew they would heal with no further intervention. It was the skin closure I was mostly concerned about.

Surface borders of the wound were so ripped and jagged they would never pull together and heal. I needed to develop cleaner, straighter lines surgically. To do that, I took a scalpel and surgical scissors and snipped away dead muscle fibers, fat, devitalized skin, all the jagged dead tissue I could. That done, I undermined the skin from its subcutaneous attachments to allow stretch without wrinkles. I was left with fresh viable edges, pliable and alive, that could be pulled together and sutured to grow into a functional scar.

Pat and I removed the bloody paper drapes we'd used to create a sterile operative field then stripped off our gloves. We deposited everything in a large, plastic trash bag. I asked Jon to see that no one touched the bloody materials and to burn them as soon as possible.

"I take care of dat," Jon said. He reached out and took the bag from me.

"Thanks, Jon," I said. "And while I have your attention, there's something else I wonder if you would do for us . . ."

Elim lies on the coastline of the Norton Sound much like Nome; but unlike Nome, it's nestled between rolling hills and valleys covered with trees. It's optimistic, calling the growths *trees* when actually, they are more like tall bushes and shrubs. But they were green and extended above ground level, giving relief to the otherwise barren Arctic landscape.

Pat wanted a Christmas tree, but there was no way to get one in Nome. I knew, with her ingenuity and motivation, she could make an Elim bush into a passable holiday decoration if only we could get a shrub back to the trailer.

"Jon, could you take my wife and me up into the hills on your snowmachine and sled to find something we can use as a Christmas tree?"

"A Christmas tree!" Pat said. "Are you kidding?"

I smiled, nodded and looked back at Jon.

"You want cut bush to use as tree?" Jon asked.

"If that's permissible."

"There no crazy law dat keep you from doing dat. And even if dere was such one stupid law, it would be white man's rule and not dat of Eskimo."

"Then let's do it," I said.

Pat clasped her palms together in an enthusiastic clap, then threw her arms around my neck and squeezed.

It was all the encouragement I needed.

We found the perfect bush-tree—especially considering our options. Jon said it was some sort of scrub pine boiled by Eskimo people to brew tea for treating arthritis. It was safe to have around children. The bush was pointed at the top and rounder at the base. With some imagination, and a bit of pruning, it could resemble the conical shape of the evergreens we'd been raised with.

Pat and I dug through snow until about four feet of the bush was exposed. Then Jon handed me his saw and I made my cut. We loaded the bush-tree up onto the sled and headed to the Elim landing strip.

Otis looked anxious. Darkness was settling in and the storm was blustering.

"We need to get this tree back to Nome," I said to Otis as he began loading our gear into the Cessna.

"It won't fit through the cargo door," Otis said. "It's frozen solid and will snap if we bend it."

I nodded. "I've got that covered." I asked Pat to hand me the sheet I wanted her to bring.

"Let's carefully fold the limbs inward to make it smaller then wrap it in this sheet. Once we've got it wrapped we'll find some string, circle it and tightened it up."

"What about using my yarn?" Pat exclaimed. She reached in her bag and pulled out a skein she was knitting into an afghan.

"Perfect!" I said.

The three of us worked the sheet around the bush-tree carefully, teasing the limbs up and inward so they didn't break. We circled the package several times with loops of Pat's yarn, cinching it up as we did.

When finished, our bundle was about the size of a large laundry bag. It fit easily through the cargo door of the aircraft and into a storage area at the rear of the plane.

It was an incredibly good feeling, improvising a tree for my family and our son's first Christmas. Though surely not the most beautiful tree we would ever have, it would certainly be the most unique and we would tell the story of its gathering to our kids for years to come.

Storm winds were building up, but we were blessed. As Otis lifted the Cessna off the rugged Elim runway, the clouds parted just enough to open a window of clear blue sky that welcomed our flight back to Nome.

PART THREE

WINTER

"Sometimes good things fall apart
so better things can fall together."
—Marilyn Monroe

CHAPTER 29

We needed a snowmachine. All right, that's a stretch. I *wanted* a snowmachine more than actually *needed* one. Money was tight, but it was getting hard to maneuver the Pontiac around mounds of snow that grew daily by the foot. Plus, snowmachines looked like fun. Every guy in town had one, and I wanted to be part of the gang.

We had saved up a little cash for a down payment, and just before Christmas I ordered a brand-new Arctic Cat Panther. About a week after it arrived, one of my patients offered to make us a real Eskimo wooden dogsled for only $125. It was a deal I couldn't pass up.

I learned the proper Arctic term for my new vehicle was *snowmachine*—not *snowmobile* as used in the lower forty-eight. That made me feel part of the community. After a couple hours training, Billy had me adept at taking the Cat with dogsled attached anyplace I felt the mood.

The doldrums of winter were taking a toll. Skies were dark when I forced myself out of bed in the morning and dark when I dragged myself home at night. I was tired all the time but slept poorly. It was irrelevant that I had no appetite since eating gave no sense of pleasure. My mind was obsessed with thoughts of work I'd left undone and mistakes I may have made. I lost my desire to have fun and even lost the joy of coming home at night to be with Pat and the kids.

At the peak of winter, the Arctic sun in Nome never rises until well after noon. Even at its fullest, it barely peaks above the horizon before slowly descending back into the sea a mere forty-five minutes later. The brief daylight the whole cycle provides casts little more than a twilight glow upon the earth, and once the twilight is gone, it's back to the blackness of night for another twenty-three hours.

One afternoon, hoping some daytime interaction with my family might lighten my mood, I sped home on the snowmachine to have lunch with Pat and the kids. After lunch, in pitch darkness driving back to clinic, an Alaska Airlines jet over headed me on its path to the Nome airport. I'd been on that flight many times and knew its route. After leaving Nome the jet would fly to Anchorage. In Anchorage, a convenient connection could be made on a Western flight that, by the end of day, would end up in Hawaii.

All I can think is . . . if I could get on that plane, in a few hours I could be in the Hawaiian Islands.

I pulled the snowmachine off the trail and watched the plane land. My mind raced with irrational thoughts. To hell with the fact I had a wife and two children. To hell with my responsibilities to the community and to the PHS. I wanted nothing more than to get on that plane and head out of Alaska to see some sun.

Out of sheer desperation, I turned the snowmachine around and headed towards the airport. About halfway there, I came to my senses. I pulled to the side of the road and burst into tears. I sobbed and sobbed, losing all physical control over my emotions. As I sat there alone in the cold bleakness of the dark afternoon crying, it began to snow, and for the first time in my life, I wondered if life was worth the struggle.

DECEMBER 23, 1971
A FEW DAYS AFTER THE WINTER SOLSTICE

We had passed the summit of winter darkness and days were getting longer by six and a half minutes every twenty-four hours. It didn't seem like much until I realized that, for every ten days, it added up to more than an hour. That was noticeable. Though I was still suffering from the condition I eventually learned was called seasonal affective disorder (SAD), the gain of daylight with every passing week started to lift my spirits.

Christmas was two days away. We wanted to make our son's first filled with memories we could share with him as he grew older: stories about his first tree we flew home from Elim wrapped in a sheet and tied with yarn, special visitors, snow, homemade gifts, and special treats he received.

We should have been careful what we hoped for.

It had been a rocky six months and Pat said we *needed* Christmas to renew our spirits; the way a dying plant needs water and sunlight. Our life had been turned upside down, living in the Arctic enduring isolation, darkness, and loneliness more than we ever thought possible. Pat felt Christmas would center us, draw us closer together as a family, and she vowed to make it the best she possibly could.

She began with the tree. Pat decorated our precious bush with origami birds that I folded from chart paper I'd brought home from the hospital. She and Chantelle colored the birds with crayons and glitter. Pat strung popcorn garlands on white yarn she was using to knit an afghan. We had no Christmas lights, so I took a table lamp and fashioned a shade of cardboard to form a spotlight we'd shine on the tree at night to make it sparkle.

Gifts, few as they were, were wrapped in heavy paper Pat bargained out of the butcher at the NC. She and Chantelle drew pictures on the paper and brought them to life with colors. Pat made bows from leftover yardage.

Christmas was on a Saturday. With clinic closed and most of our friends off work, Pat wanted to have a Christmas Day party. As newcomers to the Arctic, we could all share the day together. It wouldn't be the same as having Christmas with family, but it was better than spending it alone.

On Friday, Pat began preparations. Food was too expensive to serve a full Christmas dinner, so we decided on snacks of popcorn, nuts and a few potato chips. Most important to me was the bottle of Crown Royal I had picked up in Anchorage at a price that was way more than we could afford.

I figured the need to share a holiday drink with friends out-trumped the cost, so I rationalized the investment to be worth the money.

The party was planned for two o'clock Christmas afternoon.

I was awakened by the pitter-patter of little feet and a rumpling of blankets. When I rolled over and saw Chantelle climbing into bed with Pat and me, I thought our daughter was excited about Christmas and couldn't sleep. I was wrong.

First I heard retching. It was followed by the unmistakable sound of projectile vomit as it poured over our blankets and nightclothes. Chantelle began to cry.

"Grab a towel," Pat hollered. "Quick!"

I rushed into the bathroom and grabbed the first towel I saw. I handed the towel to Pat thinking she wanted it for cleaning up our daughter. To my surprise, it was she who filled the towel and not our poor little three-year-old.

Once Pat's retching had settled enough for her to speak, she ordered me to the kitchen to fetch a pan. When I returned, both she and Chantelle were at it again. Then I heard crying from the nursery.

"Get the baby," Pat ordered between hurls.

I handed Pat the kitchen pan and rushed to the nursery. There I found Adam in his crib, lying on his back, screaming at the top of his lungs. I picked him up and noticed he felt warm. Just as I was cradling him up to my chest, the baby heaved buckets of green bile and sour milk over my face and the front of my nightshirt. The smell was so overpowering I thought I might heave myself.

I wiped my face with the back of my hand. "It's OK, baby," I said, trying my best to comfort my son while turning my nose away from his precious little vomit-covered cheeks. I grabbed a diaper to wipe his face and mine, and he vomited again.

Ignoring the smell of the emesis, I leaned my ear against the baby's chest to listen if he was wheezing. God forbid he aspirate any vomit down into his lungs and develop aspiration pneumonia. His lungs sounded clear, but I couldn't be sure without my stethoscope and that was tucked away in my bag in the living room. I made a mental note to listen more properly when things had settled down.

"Honey," Pat hollered from our bedroom. "Is the baby OK?"

I carried Adam into the bedroom and saw Pat sitting up in a pool of vomit-soaked sheets and blankets. She was weeping and holding a crying Chantelle in her lap.

I ran back to the bathroom and brought back a fresh wet towel. I laid it over Pat's forehead.

"Better?" I asked.

She nodded, then took the towel and wiped her face and mouth.

"You feeling alright?" Pat asked me.

I'd been so busy I hadn't thought about how *I* felt until she mentioned it. And then, as if on cue, the room began to spin and my legs weakened. My stomach growled in protest as a lurch welled up into my throat. I leaned forward and grabbed the pan.

With no phone and insufficient energy to get out of the house and inform our friends the party was off, I used a crayon to scribble a note that I taped on our front door.

Sorry guys, party is cancelled.
Whole family sick as dogs.
Merry Christmas.
Tom & Pat

Our wish came true about Adam's first Christmas being memorable. It was celebrated on December 26.

CHAPTER 30

On the fourth morning after Christmas, Pat brought me a cup of coffee in bed as she had done nearly every morning since we'd been married. That morning, she included a muffin decorated with a tiny candle. With all the hustle of Christmas, our belated party and the stomach flu, I'd forgotten all about my birthday. Pat and I never once discussed any plans for the day, but that was fine. We were partied out, and the best celebration I could think of would involve nothing more than an easy day at clinic, a simple dinner with Pat and the kids afterwards, and a night filled with eight hours of undisturbed sleep.

Billy Koweluk told me the city of Nome was about to present me with a gift. He was secretive, but I thought it might be a new generator for the hospital. The gift turned out to be something even better, something more personal. A telephone for the trailer.

The phone would be installed midafternoon on my birthday and we were promised it would be in full working order by the time I got home that evening. "Full working order" meant there would be a dial tone, but that was about it. The actual telephone service would be limited to three connections—the trailer, the hospital nurses' station, and Frank Brown's home where he received calls for taxi service. I wouldn't be able to call Anchorage to consult with specialists from home, nor would I be able to give a jingle to Jamie and Billy, KNOM radio station, Alaska Airlines, or anyplace else the spirit moved me. But I was happy about getting the phone despite its limited range and thought it was moving us in the right direction towards adapting to our life in the Arctic.

I got my birthday wish about clinic. It was quick and easy. Most people in town were still in party mode awaiting New Year's Eve celebrations, and the last thing on their minds was healthy living. Many villagers were still in Nome visiting family so radio traffic was light. Those patients who did show up for clinic were truly in need of medical care and I was more than happy to take care of them.

"I'm home!" I hollered and closed the trailer door against a gush of wind. "What's for dinner?"

"Come check out the new phone," Pat said from the kitchen. "It's in the living room."

The phone was the kind of old-fashioned dial instrument from the fifties—black, no buttons or lights, and no way to place a caller on hold. It was attached to the living room wall by a curly cord long enough to stretch to both the sofa and my favorite chair. A second phone jack had been installed in the bedroom so I could move the instrument there at night.

I lifted the receiver and listened. The dial tone brought a smile to my face as I marveled at how, after six months in Nome, I'd begun to appreciate the simpler things in life.

"Dinner's ready," Pat said. "Sit down and close your eyes."

I took my usual place at our dining table. "What have you done?" I asked.

"It's your birthday dinner. What do you expect?"

"I know what I want . . . but not what I'm gonna get."

"Think again, birthday boy," Pat said, and with glee told me to open my eyes.

Sitting in front of me was a plate of my favorite meal—chicken-fried steak smothered in gravy, Minute Rice also slathered in gravy, green peas seasoned with just the slightest dab of table sugar and butter, and a bottle of Worcestershire sauce.

"How in the world . . . ?"

"It's a long story you don't need to know."

"I'm more concerned about what you paid."

"You don't need to know that either," Pat said. She pointed around the room and indicated for me to follow her finger. "You'll notice you're not getting any other presents besides this meal. So eat up and enjoy. You won't get it again for at least another year."

After dinner I read Chantelle a story, goofed around a bit with Adam, then helped Pat get the kids bathed and into bed. By eight we had the trailer to ourselves.

I was sitting on the sofa thumbing through a medical journal when a bright light poured through the living room window. The light caught my attention and I went outside to investigate its source.

The air was cold yet I hardly noticed as I stood on the trailer's front porch engulfed in absolute silence. I drew in the night and the peace that came with it. In the six months we'd been in Nome I'd never experienced an evening so . . . still. There was not the slightest hint of breeze whispering through in the air, nothing to rustle my hair or give a flush to my face. There were no sounds of engines, voices, not even the squawking of gulls that never failed to sound. The light that penetrated our window was the moon, a sliver away from being full.

The combination of the evening's still and heavy moon shot my thoughts back to San Joaquin General and the night of the rock concert. Remembering the eerie stillness of that night and the fullness of the moon chilled my spine.

A quiet night, when the air is still and the moon is full. Hospital lore holds such conditions are a setup for disaster.

I shook the memory from my head and went back inside. I wanted time to spend with my wife instead of pondering sorrows from the past.

"I feel like I should call someone," I said to Pat. "It's been so long since we've had a phone." I picked the instrument up off the floor, stretched its long cord until it reached the sofa, and sat with it on my lap.

"Call who?" Pat asked. "Installers told me the phone is only for dire emergencies and tonight we have none."

I considered what Pat said and, knowing she was right, set the phone back on the floor. I motioned for her to join me on the sofa so we could sit together in comfortable silence and simply enjoy the time. After all, it was my birthday. The night was young, and its final hours belonged to us.

That was when the phone rang for the first time.

CHAPTER 31

I was more than a little pissed. Not once had I seen my friend Garrett's wife, Juliette, in clinic for her prenatal care, yet there she was, in active labor, hauling me out on my birthday expecting me to help her. Karen Knight, a new recruit at KNOM radio station had placed her in a hospital room and was taking her blood pressure when I dragged myself in. Garrett was nowhere to be seen.

"Hasn't the public health nurse at Garrett's school been managing your pregnancy?" I asked. I slipped my parky off and tossed it over a stool. I made little effort to filter annoyance out of my voice. "I know it wasn't me."

"I told Garrett this was going to get awkward," Juliette said. She diverted her head to avoid eye contact. Her voice quivered. "Do you know MaryAnn Franklin?"

I nodded. "I've worked with her some."

"Garrett and I really wanted to do the Alaska frontier thing and have a home delivery. MaryAnn was OK with the idea, and frankly, we doubted you would be."

Juliette was right. I would not have been OK with a home delivery, especially with a first child. Home births could be hazardous. Neither would I have suggested the OB services of a public health nurse like Ms. Franklin whose specialty was immunizing kids.

"So why didn't you call MaryAnn tonight when you started labor?" I asked.

Juliette sighed and rubbed her belly. "We did, but as luck would have it, she's away for the holidays. I saw her just before she left, and everything was fine. She said she'd be back in town around the middle of January."

"I see."

"Look Tom, we wouldn't have come in at all, but I think I'm really in active labor."

"Did you and MaryAnn discuss what you would do if you went into labor while she was away?" I asked pointedly. "Garrett never said a word to me about what you were planning."

Tears welled up in Juliette's eyes and I immediately regretted the pissed-off inflection in my voice.

Put the ego aside. Just concentrate on the patient and the work.

"Not really," Juliette said. "We were just so tied up with Christmas and I guess I'm a little early."

Juliette did look very small to be full-term pregnant and in active labor, but she was still fully dressed so it was difficult to tell. I asked her to lie back and slip up her blouse so I could examine her abdomen.

Her uterus was tiny. Even to the untrained eye, she was clearly much smaller than she should be when ready to give birth.

"What's your due date?" I asked.

"MaryAnn estimated about March first based upon my last period."

"That's two months from now. Are you sure of your dates?"

Juliette frowned as a contraction began. Once it passed she said, "I was on birth control pills and my periods were erratic. Sometimes I'd go several months without one. Other times I'd have periods about every . . ." She paused as another contraction started right on the heels of the previous one. "Oh," she breathed out trying to dispel the pain. "This is rough."

"Let me feel your uterus while you have a contraction," I said. "To get a sense of how firm they are."

Juliette nodded, and I placed my hand on her belly. The next contraction peaked very firm. When it was over she asked if Garrett could come in.

"Absolutely." I said and asked the nurse to find him.

I needed a little more of Juliette's medical history and turned my attention back to her. "This is your first delivery, right?"

Juliette nodded. "And my last if it's always going to be like this. I've had morning sickness the entire time and my blood pressure has been all over the place."

"How much weight have you gained?"

"Only about six pounds. Strange because I've been eating like a pig."

"Was MaryAnn concerned about so little weight gain and your pressure?"

Juliette shook her head. "On the contrary. She complimented me on doing such a good job of staying on a diet. We never talked about the blood pressure, other than her telling me to watch my salt. I told her I never use much."

I shook my head. Pregnant women needed a healthy diet, not a calorie-restricted one. Elevated blood pressure required more attention than a cursory mention of salt usage.

Garrett stepped into the room with a smile and stood at Juliette's head. He was sipping coffee from a cafeteria mug.

"Sorry to haul you away from home, old man," Garrett said. "We didn't know what else to do."

I nodded but kept my attention on Juliette.

"Everything OK in here?" Garrett asked. "You look a little worried, Tom."

"I have some catching up to do about Juliette's pregnancy. Have a seat." I motioned toward a corner chair and Garrett sat.

I stretched a measuring tape up and down Juliette's abdomen, from her pubic bone to the top of her uterus. If she were at full term and ready to deliver, she should measure about forty centimeters. She measured only thirty-two—about right for a pregnancy seven months along. If she truly was in active labor this was not going to be good.

The thought of delivering a three-pound premature baby in the bush sent a shiver down my spine. There was no time to transfer Juliette to Anchorage and I lacked the experience and equipment necessary to deal with a preemie of that degree. Stuck out here in the wilds of Alaska, I wondered once again . . . what the hell was I going to do?

Something else about Juliette's uterus bothered me, besides its size. Not only was her womb smaller than it should be, it looked *misshapen*. Lying flat on her back, her belly should have been protuberant and uniformly round like a basketball buried under her skin. Instead, the uterus looked lumpy and oblong, wider than it was tall. I had no idea what to make of that.

"I need to do an examination that will help me determine how the baby is positioned inside your uterus," I told Juliette. "It's called a Leopold Maneuver and its done right here in the bed. You will feel a little pressure when I push on your uterus, but I promise it won't hurt you or the baby."

"Go ahead," Juliette said. Garrett stepped closer to see what I was about to do.

I placed my right hand crosswise just above Juliette's pubic bone and my left hand on her abdomen at the top of her uterine fundus. Then, applying pressure from the top, I squeezed the fingers and thumb of my right hand tightly together. Doing so, I should have been able to feel the baby's head with my right hand. I felt nothing.

"OW!" Juliette belched. "That hurts! Makes me wanna pee."

"Sorry," I said, then squeezed again a little harder. I still felt nothing, as if her pelvis was completely void of fetal parts.

Something was definitely wrong. Her strong contractions should be moving the baby down into her pelvis and the Leopold Maneuver should allow me to feel what was happening. It didn't.

Next, I palpated both lower quadrants of Juliette's uterus, pushing and squeezing as hard as she could tolerate. I closed my eyes and tried to conceptualize how the baby was lying. I felt lumps, hard areas, places I thought were parts of fetal anatomy, but they made no sense.

Another contraction came. It was very firm and lasted over a minute.

"God, I feel like I need to push," Juliette said.

"That can't be," I said. "The baby isn't engaged low enough in your pelvis to deliver. I need to check you vaginally right now!"

Juliette blinked nervously, and her lower lip began to twitch. I asked Garrett and Karen to help Juliette get out of her clothing.

I slipped on a sterile glove and started my exam. In less than ten seconds, I knew we were in for a motherlode of trouble.

Juliette's cervix was almost completely dilated, so something had to be filling the lower pelvis making delivery imminent. Yet I couldn't tell what it was or how the baby was positioned.

"I really need to push!" Juliette hollered, and just as the words blew across her lips, a gush of clear amniotic fluid exploded from her vagina.

"The baby's coming. I can feel it!"

"Membranes just ruptured!" I shouted. "We need her in the OR and into stirrups now!"

We hollered for Gracie and she, Karen, and Garrett helped Juliette scoot from the bed onto a gurney and then into the operating room. I scrubbed my hands while my two assistants lifted Juliette's legs up into cold stirrups and strapped her in.

"I've gotta push!" Juliette cried out. "It's coming."

I threw on a fresh pair of sterile gloves and slipped my hand into Juliette's vagina. To manage the birth, I needed to know the baby's presenting part. Preemies were often born breech and I wanted to be ready if that were the case.

This exam was even more confusing than my last. I felt things I shouldn't be feeling at this point; tiny parts liked curled little sausages. I didn't think they were toes because I felt nothing flat like the sole or heel. I closed my eyes. Focused. Felt again. Nothing made any sense.

"I can't help it, Tom," Juliette cried out. "I need to push."

"Do something, Tom. Please!" Garrett cried.

"Can you wait a second, Juliette? Please. Try panting."

"I can't . . . I can't. It's coming."

Juliette's swollen vaginal introitus began to spread. As she pushed, the gap widened. Horrified, I saw a trace of white skin appear in the opening.

The contraction eased and along with it Juliette's need to bear down. The patch of skin I saw momentarily retracted, but another contraction came and the drive to push was too strong for her to ignore.

Juliette cried out in pain and the white skin protruded even farther.

"Juliette, pant dammit, pant!" I begged.

Juliette tried to stop pushing but couldn't. Garrett grabbed her hand and begged her to try. She twisted her head to one side and with a muffled scream, drew her arms up over the top of her womb and grunted.

I looked down between Juliette's legs and sucked in a shocked breath. I saw something I never would have thought possible.

A tiny blue hand fell out of Juliette's vagina.

CHAPTER 32

Juliette had a rare transverse lie.

When labor started, instead of being head down as most common, Juliette's baby was lying crosswise inside her uterus. That explained why her womb looked lopsided. Because of this position, one of the baby's shoulders and arm was lying directly over the cervix when contractions began. The baby failed to rotate as it should under pressure from the contracting womb and because of that, when squeezed during labor the baby's arm stretched out to extend into the only space it could: down the birth canal. Such a presentation was vaginally undeliverable.

Transverse lie was the worst possible presentation a labor could have and damn it if it wasn't happening right here in front of me. Without a doubt, if I didn't take some affirmative action in the next fifteen minutes I'd be dealing with a catastrophic situation for *both* mother and child.

"Get Dr. Macintosh in Anchorage on a line now!" I said to Karen over Juliette's cries. "We're gonna lose this baby and mother."

I'd met Dr. Macintosh briefly during my orientation. He was chief of OB-GYN.

Karen turned and bolted from the room.

There was no time to tell Juliette or Garrett what was happening. Stout action was needed in the next few minutes or Juliette's uterus could rupture. If an immediate C-section could miraculously be performed before uterine rupture, Juliette could be saved. But there wasn't a chance in hell I could get that done before the baby died in utero.

"I have him on the line," Karen shouted from outside the room.

Thank God!

I told Gracie to stay in the room and pleaded with Juliette to try and keep from pushing while I ran to the phone. The connection was static-filled, but good enough for me to explain what I faced.

I listened intently to what Dr. Macintosh said.

"What?" I wasn't sure I heard him right. "Say again . . . "

I listened another few seconds then heard the unmistakable sound of a dial tone.

"That goddamn son of a bitch!" I screeched as I threw the phone down onto its cradle and pounded my way back to the O.R.

"What did he say?" Karen asked. She was wringing her hands and waiting for me to give her some orders.

"The bastard told me to pray. That's all he said. Pray! Then he hung up."

I cursed Macintosh's name and we dialed again. All we got in return was the dreaded repetitious tone I'd come to know that meant all phone lines were down.

"Give me a second to gather my thoughts," I told Karen. She nodded and rushed back to the OR to stay with Juliette and Gracie.

I started thinking about what would happen if I were at San Joaquin General and was faced with the same situation?

First—I wouldn't be alone. I would have a team of doctors to help me. There would be an anesthesiologist, an OB-GYN surgeon, a surgical assistant, several skilled OR nurses and techs, and a neonatologist to care for the newborn.

Second—all procedures would be done under excellent anesthesia. Anything less would be inhumane.

Third—there would be a Neonatal Intensive Care Unit with specialized nurses and equipment to watch over preemie babies like I was about to deliver.

Fourth—I had none of those things here!

Shit!

So, what would I do? I had no choice. I would improvise, be flexible, use all I learned during my internship to adapt and persevere until I got Juliette delivered. The words had become my mantra and, once again, it was time to put those principles to the test.

A scream from the OR brought me back to attention. I knew the specialist was right. Unless a miracle happened soon, prayer was the only thing that was going to help.

I closed my eyes and allowed my mind to race through a kaleidoscope of scenarios. Finally, an idea began to gel. It would be a long shot that required a lot of luck, and a miracle if it worked.

"Do we have a gauntlet sterile glove?" I asked Karen.

"I don't even know what that is," she said.

"A long glove that covers the entire forearm up to the elbow."

Karen shook her head. "If we do I've never seen such a thing."

Shit! I'll make do.

"Bring in a spinal kit."

Karen nodded and ran from the OR.

"Gracie, Garrett, help me get Juliette into a sitting position at the end of the operating table."

Gracie rushed to Juliette's side and Garrett stood.

I quickly explained to Juliette I was going to give her a spinal anesthetic and asked her to trust me. She nodded that she did.

Karen rushed into the OR with the kit and opened it with a sterile glove. I directed my attention to the lower portion of Juliette's spine.

"Lean forward a little," I said to Juliette. To Garrett, "Help hold her up and support her."

Without difficulty, I injected a calculated amount of anesthetic agent deep into Juliette's spinal canal. We waited a full minute while gravity positioned the medicine to the level I needed, then we laid Juliette down flat on her back so I could go to work.

I ripped off the sterile gloves and with one fell swoop, reached down and pulled off my shirt. Bare-chested, I hustled to the large stainless-steel sink just outside the operating room doors and began scrubbing.

"What are you doing?" Karen cried out, surprised I had removed my shirt and had fled the operating room.

"Keep watch on her BP and the fetal heart tones," I hollered back. "I'm going to do the best and highest surgical scrub I've ever done."

Using a small sponge, a brush and plenty of Betadine soap, I vigorously began debriding and washing. I used a file to clean beneath my nails then sponged and scrubbed heavily all the way up to my elbows. I rinsed, then scrubbed again, but higher this time, up to my armpits and around my shoulders and chest. Once finished, I hollered out to Karen to open the OR doors so I could come in without touching anything.

I stood there before Karen and Gracie, half naked with arms and much of my upper body covered by yellow-red soapy foam, and sighed. I was ready to do the impossible.

My plan was to reach up inside Juliette's body as far as my arm would go and snag a fetal part. Then, using whatever I grabbed I would rotate the baby to a deliverable position and drag it out alive through Juliette's birth canal.

I couldn't take a chance on donning regular sterile gloves. They came just above the wrist and when executing my plan, I would be reaching higher than that, maybe even higher than my elbows. The risk of a glove coming off during the procedure would be too great. I would have to perform the reach with a naked arm, which is why I'd removed my shirt and had scrubbed so high.

I positioned myself between Juliette's thighs and tested my spinal block by pinching a hemostat clamp on Juliette's thigh.

"Do you feel anything?" I asked.

"She's shaking her head 'no,'" said Gracie, who was seated by the operating table gently stroking Juliette's hair.

"Juliette, focus on my words now. You may feel some pressure. Try your best to hold as still as possible."

I took a second to silently bow my head and follow Dr. Macintosh's advice. In my short prayer I asked for a miracle, direction in what I was about to do. Finished with the prayer, I asked Karen to pour Betadine over my naked, ungloved arm, my shoulder and my chest. I took in a deep breath and slowly exhaled. Then, gently, as if handling the petals of a delicate rose, I cradled the tiny cyanotic hand suspended from Juliette's vagina in the folds of my palm and slowly eased my arm up into Juliette's body as far as my courage would allow.

CHAPTER 33

Reaching inside a living person's body with a naked hand and forearm was an experience that defies description. Unencumbered by latex gloves, tactile awareness of sensations on my skin were magnified tenfold—touch, temperature, moisture, pulsations. I could actually feel every beat of Juliette's heart in the tips of my fingers and appreciate the spongy texture of the placenta still keeping the baby alive. Even though I couldn't see them, my mind's eye was so acutely aware I could freely trace the trickling sensation of uterine fluids as they coursed between the lines of my palm, past my wrist and up my forearm.

Holding the baby's hand as a guide, I slowly extended my arm upward, pushing the baby back up into her womb as I went. I encountered resistance but held pressure until it faded. I reached higher, pushed farther until Juliette's vaginal opening was just inches below my elbow. It was like reaching inside a living soul.

Juliette moaned but, paralyzed from the nipple line down by my spinal block, she didn't move.

"Vitals and FHTs?" I calmly asked Karen.

"BP 110/70. Pulse 100. I haven't been able to hear the baby's heartbeat for some time."

I felt a sensation of release, as if my advancing hand had just entered a large cavity. I knew at once I had just entered Juliette's uterine space, home of the baby for the past seven months.

The baby moved. I could feel it squirm and rub against my arm as if trying to roll over. But then, in a spasmodic reflex, the baby jerked its arm and its hand slipped from my grip. I had lost my connection to the delivering child.

"Shit," I couldn't help but mutter under my breath. I needed something to hold on to, something to guide me as I blindly explored the inside of Juliette's womb. Without it, I was groping without direction.

I rotated my hand and forearm, trying to grasp some part of fetal anatomy. I moved ever so gently, fearful of rupturing Juliette's uterus or compromising the baby's umbilical cord. I felt a porous slippery surface I knew was the placenta and eased my hand away. Should I put a finger through it the resultant hemorrhage would be uncontainable. The baby would be dead in seconds.

Please God . . . Please. Guide me. It was the only thought that entered my mind. Anything more would have been an intrusion.

I felt something oblong of smooth texture, about an inch and a half long. I ran my fingers along its edge and encountered small protrusions. Digits, but smaller than the fingers of the tiny hand I previously held. I realized it was toes. I had come across a foot.

My heart skipped a beat. If I could somehow fumble about and find the other foot, I could grasp them both and pull the baby's legs down to complete the delivery as a footling breech.

I closed my eyes and tried to picture what my hand was telling me. Which foot did I feel—the right or the left? Then I thought, it didn't matter. If I could locate the great toe on the foot I held, being medial it would point the way to the other foot.

I pinched the heel of the baby's foot between my thumb and index finger, eager to keep from dropping it. Then I ran my small finger along the foot's sole picturing toes. I counted as I felt along; they were getting larger. I stretched my small finger as far as I could and located what I knew was the large toe. It was to my right side and facing upward. That told me I needed to rotate my hand counterclockwise while holding tight to the foot, and if the miracle was going to happen, a sweep of my hand would lead me to the opposite foot I needed for extraction.

The baby kicked, and damn if the foot I held didn't slip from my grip! Now I had no choice, no time to think or plan. If I didn't let instinct take over my actions, all would be lost.

Without giving it a moment's thought, I thrust my arm farther up into Juliette's uterus until my elbow was just about buried into her vagina. I rotated my arm and wrist counterclockwise as far and as high as I could. Amniotic fluid and blood flooded down my arm and the side of my naked chest and belly, but I kept exploring. I felt a knob I thought to be the heel of a foot. I grabbed it, rotated again and then felt another knob. I grabbed that. It had to be the baby's feet. Then palming both tiny feet in my trembling hand I began to withdraw my arm from Juliette's body.

"Give me fundal pressure now!" I cried to Gracie. She did. I pulled, and as I retracted my blood-soaked arm from Juliette's body out came two tiny legs through her vaginal opening.

"Stop fundal pressure," I barked the moment I had both tiny legs delivered. Gracie released her pressure, and holding both baby's legs with one hand while cradling its body with my other, I carefully lifted the child out of Juliette's birth canal.

The baby boy was not breathing. I cuddled him between my arm and chest and suctioned his nose and mouth with a bulb syringe. The stimulus was not enough to instigate a cry. I turned the baby over and held him head down so any obstructing secretions inhaled during delivery would be drained by gravity. I vigorously rubbed his back. Again, he did not take a breath.

The baby needed CPR. He was still connected to the umbilical cord, so I quickly snapped two hemostats on the cord and cut a separation. That done, I left the clamped cord dangling from Juliette's vagina and carried the baby to a nearby table. There I laid him down and began infant resuscitation.

He was flaccid and rapidly turning a dying shade of blue. I wiped his tiny nose and mouth of secretions and placed my mouth over his tiny face. I gently blew a puff of air into his lungs until I saw his tiny chest rise. I caught a break! There were no obstructions in his airway. If I could ventilate him until his own breathing instincts kicked in, perhaps he would make it.

Karen slipped a stethoscope in my ears and I listened to his tiny heart. No bigger than an acorn, it pounded strong at 140 beats a minute. I assumed his cardiac function was adequate. All he needed now was air.

I continued blowing small puffs into the baby's lungs every few seconds for a full minute. It seemed like an eternity. With each puff his chest rose and between puffs it relaxed. His dusky blue color was now turning a living shade of pink. He was alive, his heart was beating, and I was successfully ventilating his lungs. The problem was; he wasn't breathing on his own.

I paused a moment to rest. When I did, Gracie shouted that she saw the baby's chest rise on its own. I looked over, and the baby made a sputtering sound, not unlike the noise made by a clogged sink when purged by a plunger. Then he took a deep breath and grunted.

His breathing continued on its own. I listened with the stethoscope again and auscultation of his lung bases told me the lungs were clear.

"Keep an eye on him," I ordered Gracie then turned my attention to Juliette. I delivered the afterbirth easily and, upon its extraction, her uterus clamped down to a normal post-delivery size. There was no episiotomy incision to repair, no excessive bleeding to be concerned with.

Karen helped Juliette out of the stirrups and onto her bed. Juliette's body began to shake, a release of adrenaline common after stressful situations, I heard her begin to weep. Garrett was holding her hand and wiping tears from his own eyes.

I went back to Juliette's son, now wrapped in a towel by Gracie, and gathered the tiny miracle up to my chest. I looked down at the boy, no larger than a doll, and could hardly believe what had just taken place. I had reached inside a living person's body and had removed a living being. I had prayed for a miracle and now, I was holding one in my arms.

"Let me clean that little guy up and hand him to his mother," Karen said as she reached out and took the newborn from me. "You could use a little cleaning up yourself, Doc," she grinned.

She was right. My arms, chest and abdomen were covered with bodily secretions and blood that under normal circumstances would have horrified me. But at this moment, despite how despicable I must have looked, I never felt cleaner in my entire life.

Gracie came over to me and wiped down my shoulders and chest with a towel. She motioned me over to the sink and turned on the warm water so I could rest my hands under the soothing flow.

"You did really good in there, Dr. Tom," Gracie said. "I ain't never seen anyt'ing like dat in all my days."

They named the baby TJ (after me). Juliette, Garrett, and the baby stayed overnight in the hospital. I stayed with them long enough to be comfortable both mother and child were doing well, then I went home to my own family. The next morning the new parents left for Anchorage to have their three-pound, four-ounce baby checked over by a qualified pediatrician.

Two weeks later I received a letter from Garrett. TJ was in perfect health and suffered no consequences from his traumatic birth. Garrett and Juliette, however, decided not to return to Nome, agreeing they were not cut out for frontier living.

My life changed the moment I saw Juliette take the baby to her breast. I knew, without a doubt, I had found my calling in life. Despite all obstacles thrown in my path, being a doctor was the only career I could ever want. This child was not only a miracle in himself: he had created a miracle in me.

CHAPTER 34

It felt like winter would never end. Despite the small increase in daylight every day, I still felt like a prisoner to the effects of seasonal affective disorder and had no idea how to free myself from its clutches. I felt frumpy, irritable, bored. I began finding fault in meaningless infractions of everyone around me—our friends, the nurses and hospital aides, even Pat and the kids. I was so deeply exhausted at the end of each day I climbed into bed soon after dinner only to snap awake two to three hours later unable to *remain* asleep. I had responsibilities, yet wanted nothing more than to cover my head in a cave of blankets and hibernate.

I wondered if this was how my mother felt during those times when nothing brought her joy, those times when she attempted to take her life. Often, I caught myself staring out a window with a sense of detachment from my body, searching for answers to questions I didn't know how to ask. I missed my sunshine. I missed the light.

Pat suggested I keep a journal to record how much extra sunlight we got every day. It helped some, but the paltry gain of six-and-a-half minutes every twenty-four hours just didn't seem like much to get excited over.

Pat did everything she could to cheer me up. She placed few demands on me. She took care of the home, the children, even the Pontiac. She cooked my favorite meals as far as she could stretch our culinary budget.

One Saturday evening after a dinner of self-caught king crab and slaw, Pat suggested we bundle up the kids and take the Pontiac out for a drive. We seldom took the car out since there were really no places to go and the nurses always needed to be able to reach me should some emergency come in. I was content to stay home and read, but Pat insisted and I knew better than stop her when she was on a mission.

A heavy snowfall earlier in the day had camouflaged Nome and the surrounding tundra in a blanket of silvery white. The night air was quiet, pitch black, and peaceful. Clouds, now free of their moisture, had drifted far to the northeast, leaving skies overhead clear in a Milky Way of stars. I felt myself give in to the peaceful still of the night and begin to relax. Pat was right. It was exactly what I needed.

We swung by the doctor's house, our home before the trailer, and dropped in to chat with the neighbors. An hour later we said goodbye and left.

"Head out on the Teller Road a little way before we call it a night," Pat said. She added a sincere "please" that I couldn't resist

Father Poole, at KNOM radio station, had given me a small transistor radio to keep buckled on my belt. It was a way of lengthening my leash from the hospital and the trailer. Whenever I wanted to get away and was within transmission range, the DJs would call me over the air if an emergency came up and I was needed. The radio had remained silent.

I turned the car away from city lights. We drove past the hospital, past the Beltz School, and out five miles until the road became a sheet of packed snow. We drove until a patch of ice caused the Pontiac to fishtail a bit, and I considered that a sign the time had come to head back home.

"We need to turn around," I said to Pat, laying cause to the icy road.

She sighed but nodded in agreement.

I came across a small plowed turnout where I could make a "Y" turn. Just as I pulled off the main road, a curtain of bright light overtook the northern sky, rising from the horizon high into the cosmos as far as the eye could see. The light became a drape of changing color, a tapestry of gathered folds and pleats that danced and swirled like a celestial ballet. Colors in the curtain morphed from shades of green and yellow to oranges and blues, then hues of pinks, scarlet, and deep purple. It was like an artist's palette had fashioned a veil of rainbow colors that exploded into the cold night air over a background array of the star-studded night.

We'd seen the northern lights many times, but never in the shapes or hues we saw that evening. It was a magnificent sight, and though I'd never been one to consider signs or omens as anything but superstitious myth, that night I accepted the aurora as a gift, godly advice to put aside my fretful disposition and accept life in the Arctic with enthusiasm and delight. To be happy, all I need do was open myself up to the Arctic's wonders and possibilities and allow good nature to take its course.

Sitting there in the Pontiac, my mood lightened as if a cloak had been lifted from my shoulders. I looked over at my wife, her face aglow from the shining lights, and smiled for the first time in days.

We sat in the comfortable quiet of the car and simply enjoyed the time together until the glorious lights of heaven faded away. Then I drove home, a different man than when we'd left.

CHAPTER 35

T he morning temperature lingered at subzero, yet the sun was so bright and the air so clear, I thought the day should be granted an award. I'd never seen a sky so blue and air so free of pollution. The moment I stepped outside and inhaled the day's freshness, I made a vow our kids would grow up in a place where we couldn't see, smell, or taste the air we breathed.

It was a Sunday. KNOM was broadcasting soft, easy listening music and not once had my name been called out for an emergency. I had made hospital rounds early and radio traffic had taken less than an hour. Unless something unforeseen happened, I would have the rest of the day completely free.

"Eric Rodgers is the DJ this morning," Pat said. "He just announced we'll have about five hours of full sun today. Why don't we call a couple of people and have a winter picnic?"

"It's below freezing outside."

"You always say people can dress for the cold."

"Yeah, but it's *really* cold."

"Come on. Let's drop by the radio station and see if Helen and Don are free. We can take the snowmachine and sled out toward the Roadhouse and watch the ocean."

"The ocean's frozen," I reminded Pat.

"Don't be such a kill joy. I'll throw together some sandwiches, maybe some hot cocoa, and we can enjoy the few hours of sunshine."

The thought *was* appealing. I couldn't remember the last time I had felt any sun on my face.

"You get lunch ready and the kids taken care of. I'll connect the dogsled to the Cat and check our fuel."

Pat gave me a welcomed hug. "You got it," she said, and went to work setting up a feast.

We dressed in layers of cotton and wool and bundled up in our parkys. Pat plastered sunscreen on both the kid's faces and took time to safety pin Adam's mittens to the sleeves of his tiny blue snowsuit. We got to the rectory around 11:00 and didn't need to convince Helen and Don to join us.

"Can I hold Adam for the ride?" Helen asked.

Pat smiled and nodded. "He's squirmy, so you'll need to hold on to him tight."

"I'll consider it hugs," Helen said.

Don helped Helen snuggle up inside our fur-lined reindeer sleeping bag and they both took their places on the dogsled. Once seated, Don pushed back to the musher's handrail and Helen huddled in between his legs.

"You ready for Adam?" Pat asked.

Helen gave Pat a thumb's up and Pat handed her our son.

Helen carefully tucked Adam tightly between her knees and I took my usual seat at the driver's position. Pat sat behind me with Chantelle stuffed between us.

Settled in place, I turned around to check with Helen and Don. Their smiling faces, peeking out between the edges of the fur bag, told me they were ready to go. I fired up the powerful machine, and off we sped into a day of sun, fun, and relaxation.

The Roadhouse, a seedy bar and steakhouse about twenty miles east of town, served beer and wine, over-priced sinewy steaks, salad, and baked potatoes. The place bellied up to the road across from the Bering Sea coastline and sported a nice porch we thought we'd use while wolfing down our sandwiches.

To get to the Roadhouse from Nome, patrons drove along a highway that paralleled the beach. The road came so close to the ocean in places that even the slightest deviation off-trail could send a traveler deep into a plowed snowdrift; or worse, through a crack in the frozen sea to meet a watery death.

A heavy snow had plummeted down on the area the night before and heat from vehicles driving on the road eventually pounded the fresh powder to a slick, glazed sheet of ice. Even though ocean breakup was months away, a narrow strip of water had opened up along the shoreline as a reaction to radiant heat from the high Arctic sun. A glare caught my eye, momentarily blinding me, and I jolted. The jar caused the snow machine to lurch, then veer abruptly to the right. If I didn't correct the misdirection quickly, we would plunge right into the churning water and ice floes of the ocean. I reacted out of instinct, sharply twisting the Cat's handlebars back to the left, but I corrected too hard. The snowmachine shimmied and went into a spin.

"Watch out!" Pat screamed. But it was too late.

I felt the rear of the snowmachine shudder then twist as it lifted off the trail. I jerked my head around and saw the dogsled with our precious cargo rise up into the air, shake, then slam down with a crash. We spun faster, and the sled lifted again, higher now, to crash down a second time.

I tried to stop, but applying the brake caused the spin to accelerate. I throttled to dampen the spin, but the Cat shot forward in a blast of uncontrolled power. The spin accelerated even harder and I felt the rear of the snowmachine shudder again and rise off the roadway. This time, I heard a tearing sound like metal scratching against metal and a hard thwack. I jerked my head around to check the dogsled and was horrified by what I saw.

My mind recorded it in slow motion. The dogsled had ripped away from its attachment to the snowmachine and was catapulted into the air upside down. I saw arms and legs splay out from under the reindeer sleeping bag as the sled crashed down against the frozen road. Screams filled the air as the sled hit, rolled twice, then skidded to a stop on its side. I heard Helen shriek and Don holler to ask if she was OK. Then, I saw a tiny, light blue snowsuit eject from under the rumbled sled and skid along the frozen pathway—twenty, thirty feet. It left a bloody trail in its wake.

"The baby!" Helen screeched through a tangle of coats, fur, and crumbled wooden debris. "I've dropped the baby."

I killed the snowmachine motor and checked that Pat and Chantelle were OK. They were frightened, but without injuries. I bolted off the snowmachine and headed for my son.

When I got to Adam he was lying perfectly still, face down on the ice in a rapidly enlarging circle of blood. He was not crying. The silence stopped my heart.

I swooped up my son and gathered him to my chest. I cradled his tiny head to support his neck, God forbid he'd suffered a cervical fracture that would render him a quadriplegic. I spun his body around so I could see his face. It was a sheet of frozen blood. His mittens had ripped off and lay dangling from his parky sleeves where Pat had pinned them. Both his little bare hands were now a mass of bleeding cuts.

My baby appeared stunned, but not unconscious. I could tell by flares of his nostrils and heaves of his chest, he was breathing. I quickly unzipped his parky and slipped a finger to the side of his neck. There was a pounding carotid pulse, regular and strong, fast as I would expect after a traumatic injury.

After a moment, Adam whimpered then opened his eyes. When he recognized me, he reached his arms around my neck and let out a blood-curdling cry. It was the best sound I had ever heard.

I attempted to assess his injuries on the frozen ground, but I was too emotional to do anything productive. All I could tell was that he was moving his head and all extremities, his heart was beating and he was breathing. A more in-depth exam would have to wait until we got to the hospital and Jamie could get some X-rays.

I wiped the blood from his little face and hands with my shirt. Then I unzipped my own parky, brought him to my chest, and stuffed him inside. If he slipped into shock, the best thing I could do was keep him warm.

Helen and Don were shaken, but not injured. Helen was far more concerned about Adam than herself. She was nearly hysterical, crying, apologizing that she'd dropped him when the sled crashed. I reassured her it was not her fault.

Don and I pulled the tattered dogsled off the road and left it on its side. God forbid our debris would cause another accident and someone to get hurt.

"Get him to the hospital and don't worry about us," Don said. "Someone will come along and take us home. If not, we can walk."

I nodded and jumped on the Cat with Adam bundled inside my coat. I motioned to Pat to grab Chantelle and join me. With one adrenaline-infused pull of the starter rope, the snowmachine burst to life. Carefully, slower than I had ever driven before, we made our way back toward town.

We spotted Frank Brown in his taxi. I told him what happened and asked him to go fetch Jamie first then head out toward the Roadhouse to pick up Helen and Don. Frank had Jamie at the hospital only moments after we arrived ourselves.

I would have given anything to have had some other physician step in and take over my son's care. But there was no one to help, no one with experience or training to do what was necessary to check him over. It had to be me. I had to separate myself emotionally from my child to become his doctor. It was a task no physician father ever wanted to face.

I actually felt a change come over me. I detached all emotion from my baby, wiped my eyes of tears, washed my hands, and diverted focus away from everything in the room except the need to take care of my child.

The first thing I did was place a brace of rolled towels around his neck until X-rays could be taken. Once Jamie's films determined that no fractures had occurred, I removed the homemade brace and went on to examine every part of my child's tiny body. I took my stethoscope and listened to his heart and lungs, rotated every joint, examined every major muscle group, pushed and prodded his belly and felt every area of soft tissue on his entire frame. I examined every inch of his skin for cuts and tears.

His face and hands were frostbitten and badly abraded. His eyes were clear and all neuro checks and reflexes were normal. Every joint, every bone seemed perfectly intact. His belly was soft and lungs abundantly full of air as he cried hysterically the entire time. All in all, it was a miracle he wasn't hurt more seriously.

The cuts, scratches, and ice burns on his skin would heal. Only one small laceration on his forehead required sutures, and I took particular care in closing it with hopes it would heal without scarring. I prayed any injuries to his psyche would heal just as well as I knew his body would.

Once my examination was complete and I was confident Adam was not seriously injured, I wrapped him in a hospital gown and covered him with a blanket. He had cried himself to sleep by the time I handed him over to his mother.

Now I could relax, give up my robotic poise, and become his dad again. My hands, steady while I was the examining physician, began to tremble, as did my lower lip. My eyes clouded over with tears as my mind fogged with thoughts of what could have happened.

It was more than I could bear. I excused myself from Pat, the nurse, Jamie, and everyone in attendance, and slipped outside for a moment alone. I stood there, lost in a kaleidoscope of thoughts and images. As the last of the day's sunshine sank below the western horizon, I vomited over the freshly fallen snow.

CHAPTER 36

My relationship with the acting hospital administrator Mr. Harland McCoy was not going well.

I'd never had issues with authority figures, so that wasn't the problem. I understood the principle of relating to authority was respect for the *uniform*—not the person themself. What I didn't understand was how McCoy thought he had any authority over me.

I took orders from the Service Unit Director in Kotzebue, who took orders from Anchorage, and so forth up the chain of government hierarchy until it reached that ultimate one, POTUS. McCoy, on the other hand, considered himself my *boss* and that caused problems.

Whenever McCoy and I engaged in conversation that resulted in differing opinions, we had a relentless way of butting our heads together until one of us exploded in anger. I knew it was more than just *personality* conflicts. The growing animosity between us came down to one simple fact: he represented the private sector of healthcare and I represented the government's.

Miss Lydia Green was the town's busybody. She was the type of person who enjoyed creating trouble even if there was none to be found. Lydia was in her midseventies, had flaming red hair that required touching up once a month, and a scarlet personality that matched her hair color.

I knew Lydia by reputation but had never met her in person. I certainly had never seen her in clinic. If she were ill, she'd be the first to head directly to the airport rather than the hospital to be seen by a "government doctor."

One day, I received a letter from Dr. Hayden in Anchorage, asking me to respond to a letter of complaint he had received from Lydia Green about my work in Nome. The letter, and the complaints it referenced, were endorsed and supported by none other than the hospital administrator, Mr. Harland McCoy.

I was accused of three transgressions:

First, I was blamed for failing to diagnosis acute appendicitis in a fifty-year-old man named Thomas O'Brian. According to Miss Green, Mr. O'Brian presented to my clinic with classic right lower quadrant pain with vomiting for which I diagnosed food poisoning. The letter went on to say that, fortunately, the man visited another physician who promptly made the correct diagnosis and took Mr. O'Brian to surgery where his life was "saved by the skin of his teeth by a physician who knew what he was doing."

Next, I was accused of prescribing the wrong antibiotic for a woman suffering from pneumonia. Miss Green's letter stated that Emma Skies was highly allergic to penicillin. I, supposedly, was aware of her allergy yet prescribed the drug for her anyway. According to Miss Green, had Emma taken just one of the pills I'd given, she would have suffered anaphylactic shock and died.

Third, Miss Green brought up the issue of Jessie Clark, the boy with the fractured arm. Her letter stated the boy had not been seen nor examined quickly enough when brought in the hospital, and he was left alone, on a stretcher, suffering extreme pain while other, less emergent patients were being treated.

Dr. Hayden instructed me to respond immediately to Miss Green's allegations as time was of the essence. Because the charges were so severe, the commander said, were I not able to satisfactorily explain each case away, I'd be subject to severe disciplinary action that could include court marital and possible imprisonment.

I began my defense research by searching my clinic files for a patient named Thomas O'Brian, the man in whom I allegedly misdiagnosed acute appendicitis. The name wasn't familiar, and I found no such records under that name. Pat went to work, and after much digging did find a Mr. O'Brian—but I had never seen him for *any* medical condition, let alone, abdominal pain. It turned out the diagnostic error had been made at a clinic in Seattle when the man had gone to the lower forty-eight on a shopping spree with his wife. On his way back home to Alaska, O'Brian's abdominal pain worsened so he and his wife stopped off in Anchorage where appendicitis was diagnosed and an appendectomy was appropriately performed.

Emma Skies was an unusual name. I knew I would remember it, but I could not recall ever seeing such a patient in clinic or the hospital. As with Mr. O'Brian, a search of medical records failed to produce any written documents I ever did. Since the compliant referred to a prescription, I made a visit to Nome Pharmacy to discuss the case with my friend and local pharmacist, Ed Greenberg.

"I remember the case very well," Ed told me. "Emma Skies."

Ed continued. "Emma saw a doctor in Anchorage who prescribed her Keflex. When she came into the pharmacy to have it filled, I had down in my records she was penicillin allergic. Since Keflex is chemically related to penicillin and sometimes can cross-react with it, I suggested Emma call the doctor in Anchorage and get a different Rx."

"Then it's not my name on the prescription?" I asked Ed.

Ed shook his head and showed me the written prescription he had on file. Printed clearly below a scribbled signature was the name: Dr. Mark Fields, MD, Internal Medicine, Anchorage, Alaska.

Jessie Clark. I remembered the boy well and his father. I also remembered that at the time Jessie came into the hospital I had a baby crowning and an appendectomy in progress when the power went out. Jessie had been attended to properly by my assistants upon my orders. He had been made comfortable with the proper type and dose of pain medication and was told I would get to him just as quickly as I could.

The boy knew I had two serious patients ahead of him and he understood his need to wait.

I spent every free moment the next three days drafting a letter to Dr. Hayden. Once I had discovered all the facts about each complaint I became furious that McCoy had not done the same. I could not understand why he was so quick to join with Lydia Green in causing grief with my superiors in Anchorage, but I sure as hell wanted to find out.

When I asked McCoy about the cases and why he didn't look into them before forming an opinion, he refused to answer. Instead, he hid behind the veil of not being allowed to discuss a case that was under investigation.

Two weeks later, I received a letter from Anchorage that a full inquiry had been conducted and absolutely no fault was found. No disciplinary action against my work or me would be taken and each case would be dismissed.

I never received an apology from McCoy or any word from Lydia Green. But my heart labored over what happened, wondering why I was so disliked, why someone would want to hurt me so.

The incident was a turning point for my life and work in Nome. It helped me to come to one important conclusion I'd been shoving to the back of my mind. I was starting to think about getting out of Nome. Permanently.

CHAPTER 37

I was sitting at my office desk enjoying a cup of coffee before starting clinic when I noticed an envelope from administrator McCoy.

I never knew what to expect from the hospital administrator, except that it was seldom good. Ever since the incident with Lydia Green, McCoy had avoided contact with me, a behavior that suited me fine. I considered waiting until day's end to see what he wanted, but I'm a glutton for punishment and decided to open his note.

His memo was short and to the point. I was to come by his office immediately upon arriving at clinic and definitely before starting with patients. There was no "please" in his request, no "thank you" or indication he would appreciate a moment of my time. Just a command . . . and to make it snappy.

I glanced at the clock on my office wall. The first patient would arrive in fifteen minutes. I decided to give McCoy ten.

"Go right in," Regina said timidly with eyes planted on her desk. It was her tell that meant something unpleasant was up. "He's expecting you."

I tapped on the door and heard a grunt I assumed was my cue to enter. "You wanted to see me?"

"Come in," the administrator said.

"I've got about ten minutes. Heavy schedule today. It's Tuesday." My schedule wasn't heavy but I didn't want this meeting to drag on.

"Take a seat," McCoy instructed me. "I have some news."

"About?"

"I have something for you," McCoy said. He reached across his desk and handed me a sealed envelope. "Read its contents carefully when you have time. It's very important."

"How about you tell me now," I said.

McCoy grinned. I knew something was up.

"Run along now, please. I'm a busy man. I think the notes will make themselves perfectly clear."

I just couldn't resist opening the envelope the moment I got back to my office.

Inside were two notes. The first informed me that a nurse from Seattle—Leona Perone, RN—had been hired to become the hospital's new director of nursing. She would be in charge of all nursing staff, protocols, and schedules. Sally, who had held the position for over two years, would be relieved of her duties the moment Miss Perone arrived. I was advised that any hospital policies that involved direct patient care were to be run directly through Miss Perone and that I was to take orders directly from her.

Fat chance of that happening!

The second note was an invoice, made out to Mr. and Mrs. Thomas Sims. It was for services rendered by the hospital for obstetrical care given to one Mrs. Patricia Sims for the birth of an infant son. I had to laugh out loud. One item on the bill was a charge for $400 listed as "physician's services." The son of a bitch was trying to charge us for *my* work as the physician who delivered his own child!

I crumbled up both sheets and tossed them into the nearest trash container.

CHAPTER 38

L eona Perone, the new director of nursing, could have been the poster
model for an advertising campaign seeking military nurses. She wasn't
military; she was old school—of an era in which nurses ran hospitals the
way nuns ran convents and doctors were one step down from God.

Nurses like Leona actually *stood* when a doctor entered the room and
called doctors "sir" when in their presence. She treated me that way, and
it made me most uncomfortable. One of the first conversations I had with
Leona revolved around our working relationship. I asked if I might call her
Leona, and suggested she call me Tom. She frowned, said she appreciated
the gesture, but would only be comfortable if I addressed her as Nurse
Perone or Miss Perone, and I certainly would be nothing less to her than
Dr. Sims.

Every day, Nurse Perone looked the same; a staunch middle-aged lady
with gray-streaked hair pulled so tightly into a bun I thought her face must
ache. Her dress was always a white hat, white uniform, white stockings,
white shoes, and a white watchband wound around a pasty white, skinny
wrist. Even her well-manicured fingernails were painted a pasty white
like those of a corpse. Her skin was so pale, were it not for the icy blue of

her eyes and the few remaining streaks of brown in her hair, I could have mistaken her as albino.

Leona hit the hospital like a Midwest tornado. She flitted down the hospital hallways instead of walking, her uniform so stiffly starched it moved in unison with every breath she took. She spent her days opening cabinets and closets, sifting through drug supplies and bandages, inspecting each of the six patient rooms. She was never without a clipboard, always taking names, making notes, asking people their position in the hospital system. It took less than a week for everyone, except McCoy and me, to despise her.

The first nail in Leona's coffin was the powerhouse manner in which she took control of every department in the hospital. She lived by rules, codes of conduct and dress, all of which she claimed were designed to make the hospital a more professional institution. When she disagreed with the way an area was handled, she accused the person in charge of knowing nothing about nursing services, nothing about patient care, and nothing about running a team of professionals skilled in the delivery of medical care.

I actually liked Leona. I appreciated her enthusiasm for the job, her energy to get things done in a hospital that really needed it. I trusted her takeover mannerism would settle down once she got into the spirit of the hospital and appreciated the overall feeling of family all of its employees enjoyed. I was wrong.

It took just a week for Leona to completely revamp every nursing protocol the hospital had. The alliance she formed with Administrator McCoy was so strong, he allowed her to make changes in every department of the hospital she wanted, save one notable exception—the combined X-ray and lab run by Queen of the Hospital, Jamie Koweluk. Jamie made it perfectly clear: mess with her and she was gone. Everyone, including McCoy, knew the hospital would fall apart should that ever happen.

Sally was the first of Leona's victims. Overnight she was demoted to floor nurse and assigned the worst nursing job in the hospital: night shift. Helen and Connie threatened to quit after she told them how to dress, how to administer medications, how to set up the OR, the emergency area, even hospital rooms and the newborn nursery—areas they'd been handling perfectly well for over a year. Thankfully, both stayed, but only after I begged. Leona even had the gall to take on Esther and Gracie, foundations of patient care for over a decade. Humbly, the two bowed their heads and condescended to every command the new nursing director issued.

After a month, Sally could no longer take the stress of working under Leona. One night she failed to come in for work. Leona contacted every nurse on staff, seeking coverage for the night, but when every single one fabricated an excuse why they couldn't make it in, Leona had to take the midnight shift herself. It sent her into a rage.

The following day, we learned that Sally had taken an Alaska Airlines flight to Anchorage and had left Nome for good. We would never see her again.

Everyone loved Sally and the news of her departure echoed throughout the community like wildfire. It would be the start of a war; a conflict between myself, McCoy, and Leona Perone that would have serious repercussions on my relationship with the MMM Hospital and my life and work in Nome.

CHAPTER 39

I loved how the April sun peeked over the foothills east of Nome in the early morning and didn't set at night until close to nine. On such a day a person could bundle up, stand outside under brilliant skies and freezing temps, and allow the heat from the northern sun to tickle the senses.

Sixteen-hour days were a blessing and a curse. On the plus side, longer days helped my winter depression fade and provided more time for clinic where numbers increased with every passing week. On the minus, longer days gave residents more time to fish and hunt, which meant more opportunities to hit a bottle, get injured, and fall into trouble.

At 8:15 a crowd had already begun to gather for clinic. I decided to get an early start and had just stepped into an exam room when Helen burst through the door and grabbed me by the sleeve.

"You've gotta get downstairs to the radio room," Helen ordered. "There's an emergency call from Golovin."

"What's happening?" I asked Helen.

"Transmission is garbled but I think the health aide is worried about a woman in labor."

Crap! That really wasn't good. My first week in Nome I discovered that Eskimo women rarely had problems delivering babies. I believed it was because natural selection had worked miracles over eons of time so that typical labor in Eskimo women, even for a first delivery, lasted only about an hour and was never accompanied by a whimper. My colleagues from the lower states never believed it when I told them that, but it was true. I figured, if a Golovin woman was having trouble and she was crying out in pain, the situation brewing could be serious.

I excused myself from my clinic patient and ran down the stairs to the radio room.

"This is KIC-736 Nome Hospital calling KMM-426 Golovin," I shouted into the microphone. I always spoke loudly when anxious. "Come back, Golovin. This is Dr. Sims. Do you have a copy?"

The radio sprung to life in broken syllables. "This is KM . . .426 . . . olovin. Com . . . n . . . over."

"I copy, Golovin, but transmission is not clear. Is this Lois?"

The damned radio hissed like a snake. "Roger, Doctor. This is Lois Arrluk. I have . . . year o . . . nine months preg . . . pain."

Her next words made me nervous. "Heavy . . . cramp . . . bleeding . . ."

It didn't take a specialist in obstetrics to know the situation was grim. Cramping and bleeding at this late stage of pregnancy usually meant one of two things: abruption or placenta previa. Both could be life threatening—to both the newborn and mother.

Golovin was seventy air miles away. There was little I could advise the health aide to do other than have her place the laboring mom on her left side. To save this mother and child, my best hope was to hightail it out to Golovin as quickly as a plane could get me there, and pray nothing tragic happened before I arrived.

I asked Helen to get me a charter with Munz Northern and Esther to hustle up Frank for transport to the airport.

"Frank in cafeteria having coffee with Gracie," Esther said with a toothless grin. "They been dating after she break up with dat damn Ben Aracutuk."

"OK," I shouted. "I'm off. I'll be in touch."

I ran down to the cafeteria and on the way grabbed my parky and a small medical go-bag I kept for emergencies. I found Frank sitting at a table with Gracie, laughing. When Frank saw the panic in my eyes he knew I needed him. "Taxi, Doc?" he asked.

"You bet," I said. "Airport, pronto. I'll give you details on the way."

As we sped down the icy road I realized I hadn't thought to have someone contact Pat to let her know I was leaving. I shrugged the feeling off, thinking it shouldn't be a problem. I'd be back home and ready for lunch before she ever knew I was gone.

Otis sat at the controls of the Cessna 180, prop spinning and cabin warming. He waved us over the moment Frank pulled up.

"Got something big going on in Golovin?" Otis asked.

I nodded. "We better step on it or there's a chance we could lose both a mother and a baby."

"That's all I need to know, Doc."

Otis reached down, grabbed the few things I'd taken out of Frank's cab, and helped me settle into the front seat next to him. I held the go-bag on my lap.

I clicked my seat harness into place and Otis gave it a tug. He smiled, then pushed the Cessna's throttle to full thrust and the tiny airplane shuddered in response. The plane spun around, and in a gust of blowing snow, headed toward the end of the Nome runway.

CHAPTER 40

Visibility was bleak. Low, thick weather rich clouds had drifted in from the sea overnight and blanketed the area with heavy fog and blowing sleet. It wasn't my favorite type of flying weather.

"You gotta know, Doc, flying's going to be touch and go today," Otis said. "We'll be IFR the entire way."

My breathing quickened. I knew IFR meant Instrument Flight Rules—a fancy way of saying visibility was poor and flying would be done using instruments. I hated IFR flights. From my perspective, IFR meant only one thing: WSFD, my own acronym for Weather Shitty, Flying Dangerous.

Otis looked over at me and grinned. He knew I was a big jet kind of guy. Normally I took my share of teasing when forced to fly in less than perfect air, but Otis seemed to realize I was in no mood for razzing, so he didn't make jokes.

"You get air sick?" Otis asked.

"Not yet."

"Well if you don't get it this trip, you never will. Now hold on tight, Doc. This is gonna be a hoot."

As Otis predicted, the plane pitched and rolled for the next hour. I suffered nausea, but the feeling was trumped by the ache in my hands as I white-knuckled my seat armrest the entire flight.

We buzzed the village—a standard practice bush pilots used to alert residents a plane is coming in—then Otis made his signature butter-smooth touch down on the icy landing field without incident. I was relieved to have kept the contents of my breakfast inside my gut, but my hands were so numb I prayed I wouldn't need them for anything technical until I had a chance to rub them back to life.

I spotted two men on snow machines approaching from the village. Otis motioned for me to open my cabin door and climb out, but he didn't join me nor did he cut the Cessna's engine. As soon as my feet touched the snow-covered ground, Otis reached over and handed me my medical bag.

"I gotta get right back to Nome," Otis shouted over the roar of the deafening wind. "It's almost whiteout conditions now and this storm's gonna be a humdinger. Have someone radio our office when you're ready to come home."

"Can't you wait until I check things out?" I said. I certainly did not want to remain stranded in Golovin any more than Otis did.

"Sorry, Doc, I'd really like to, but I can't."

Just then a bolt of lightning sliced across the sky, followed by a roar of thunder that nearly knocked me off my feet.

"I'll get back to pick you up just as soon as you call. Best I can do, Doc."

"But the radio doesn't work half the time and it's on generator. Can't you . . ."

Before I could finish, Otis pulled the cabin door shut. He revved the engines and the plane turned in a burst of blowing snow. Within seconds the Cessna was racing down the runway and the last I saw of it, it was being swallowed up by a cloak of dank black clouds.

There I was: alone and stranded in Golovin, Alaska—a tiny village perched on a spit of land that jutted out into a bay off the Bering Sea. The only items I had with me were a jacket and a small medical bag. The village had no electricity except for a few scattered generators, no phones, no way to communicate with the outside world except an antiquated radio that belched and shivered with every change in the weather. And the storm of the century was on its way.

I wondered how bad this was really going to get.

Blood and amniotic fluid saturated the bed and much of the floor of the young woman's hut. Clutter was scattered everywhere, but I was relieved to see there was no dead baby lying in its midst. The mother-to-be looked about nineteen, heavy set, and frightened. I noticed she had lighter skin tones and hair color than most Eskimo women her age, but I made nothing of its importance at the time. She was lying on her left side as I had advised and was sweating profusely. The village health aide, Lois Arrluk, was hovering over her, wiping her brow and massaging her temples. Several older women were gathered around, singing and humming spiritual songs. There were no men inside the hut.

"What's your name?" I asked the young woman. I placed my hand on her belly to feel the height of her uterus.

"Susan," she muttered between short, uneven breaths. Her eyes squeezed shut as her face grimaced with the tightening of another contraction. She cried out in pain when it peaked.

Once the contraction passed I asked Susan to roll flat on her back for examination. I draped a blanket over her legs and told her to lift her knees.

"Bend your knees," I instructed Susan when she lifted them off the bed. "Let them to fall apart so I can look at you more closely."

Her inner thighs and pubic region were stained with the same foul mixture of blood and brown fluid that stained her bed. I leaned closer and was met with an oddly sweet odor. It wasn't urine. It was meconium—amniotic fluid that bathed the infant inside the uterus but was now stained with infant stool. The fluid had escaped the uterus and flooded the bed when her water broke. Meconium-stained amniotic fluid was a bad omen. It meant the baby was in distress and must be delivered soon.

I paused a moment to consider what to do next. I took a deep, solid breath and shook my hands to dispel their cramping.

First, I needed to know if the baby was still alive. That itself presented a challenge since the only listening device I had at my disposal was a nearly useless regular stethoscope.

I placed the bell of my stethoscope on Susan's abdomen and listened intently. Nothing.

"Could you please stop singing for a moment?" I asked the women circling Susan's cot. "If we can all keep it very still for just a moment I might be able to hear something."

The women all shushed one another. Several actually held their breath. Two women grasped hands while another made the sign of the cross over her chest and face.

I waited until another contraction passed, then readjusted the placement of my stethoscope, lower this time and to the right side of Susan's belly. I closed my eyes and held my breath.

There it was—a soft ticking sound running about 140 taps per minute. The baby was still alive.

"How long has she been in labor?" I asked Lois.

"Long time. Maybe five, six hours now."

It was too long for a typical Eskimo woman's labor and she was in too much distress. I needed to discover what was wrong. I needed to perform a vaginal exam.

"Lift your legs again, Susan, and let your knees fall apart like you did before."

She shook her head no, muttering she was afraid and embarrassed.

"Do it!" I grunted. Time was running short. This baby was in big trouble and needed to be delivered in the next few minutes. I glanced over to Lois and with a nod of my head asked her to help.

"Come on, honey," Lois said to Susan. "You need do as doctor says. He good man and here to help."

Lois reached down, lifted both of Susan's knees and pushed them apart.

"I could use more light," I said into the room.

One of the chanting women grabbed a kerosene lantern off a table and carted it over to the bedside. I pointed between Susan's legs. "Try to direct some light here."

The woman did as I asked, dangling the lantern between Susan's parted knees and my face.

The lantern helped. I could see the opening of Susan's vagina, bulging as if under extreme pressure, but there was no sign of a delivering baby.

"Pour some of this iodine solution over my hand and Susan's birth canal," I instructed Lois as I pulled on a sterile glove.

Lois did as I asked.

"Try to relax," I said to Susan. "I'm going to wait until you have another labor pain, and then I'm going to check inside you right while you're having the contraction."

My thoughts drifted back to San Joaquin General, when just a few months before I had waited for patients in labor to have a contraction so I could check them. I was amazed at the difference in the situation now. At San Joaquin General I had everything needed to insure a good result. Here in Golovin, all I had was my examining hand and a camping lantern to light my way.

Susan moaned as her belly tightened. The moment the contraction reached its peak I slipped my gloved hand deep into her vagina in order to explore. Susan complained and batted at me, but I persisted. I held hope that whatever was halting the progress of her labor would literally be at my fingertips. With that, I'd be able to set a plan into action that would get this child delivered.

I closed my eyes and focused. I probed, reached, and twisted, feeling for pelvic landmarks and soft parts in the baby's skull—fontanels—that would help me determine the size of Susan's pelvis and how the baby was lying inside the womb.

The contraction relaxed, and I withdrew my hand. I sighed and drew in a deep breath. With a sinking heart, I had discovered the problem and it filled me with fear. I had no idea how to handle it.

Odds were stacked heavily against us for a good result. This was Susan's first pregnancy, she was overweight, and her baby was huge. She was also bleeding, and the meconium staining of her amniotic fluid told me the baby was in trouble. On pelvic exam I'd determined Susan had a small pelvis compared to other Eskimo women I had delivered, and that would make delivery difficult. The reason for her pelvic issue came to me quickly. Genetics.

Susan was of mixed race—Caucasian and Eskimo. It was why her skin was light in color and why her pelvis small compared to other, full blooded

Eskimo women. Added together, all the problems I saw with getting Susan delivered were serious, but they paled compared to one thing that was worst of all. Susan's her baby was coming down the birth canal area breech.

Breech deliveries are dangerous to both mother and child, especially with first pregnancies. It is the reason most breeches are delivered by cesarean section. I could do a C-section in Nome, but in Golovin, performing the procedure was virtually impossible. I had to think of something else.

I made a mental inventory of what I had and what I didn't.

Obviously, there was plenty I *needed*: anesthesia; scalpels; suture material; an umbilical cord clip; sterile surgical instruments; forceps, needles and syringes; dressings; IV fluids; medications to stop bleeding; oxygen; isolette for the newborn; diapers. All the normal things a hospital supplies for mothers about to have a child.

What I had was: two pairs of sterile gloves; Betadine soap; a bundle of Band-Aids held together by a rubber band; a couple of syringes, but no helpful medicines to use with them; scissors that were not sterilized; and my stethoscope. It was an "up shit creek without a paddle" scenario and I knew it.

I closed the medical bag and stared out into the room. I had to pull myself together and think. What did we do at San Joaquin General that affected a positive outcome when we had obstetrical problems? What had I learned that could get me through this without suffering a major loss?

Nothing in my training ever came close to preparing me for what confronted me now. I had to think outside the box, come up with a plan for which my training *hadn't* prepared me.

I remembered an amusing technique I'd learned in medical school during my OB rotation. It was told to me, not by one of my professors, but by a lovely grandmother who was sitting with her thirteen-year-old granddaughter laboring with her first baby.

"Birth canal gonna be small in young girl like this," the grandmother said, patting the girl's hand as she cried through every contraction. "My

Ellie is just a baby herself," the grandmother complained. "Babies havin' babies. Lord have mercy, it just ain't right but that's the way it is these days."

I nodded that I understood.

"You know, Doc, this little child of mine is gonna have a problem if you don't do somethin' special. Her little baby vagina is just too tiny to pass out a livin' child. You gotta make that honey spot of my baby girl open up further so that young'un of hers come out the way God intended."

I couldn't hold back my smile at her descriptive language: honey spot, babies havin' babies. I felt honored she trusted me with terms she clearly understood.

"You gotta do pussy massage, Doc. That's what it's gonna take. Good old pussy massage."

"What exactly do you mean?" I asked.

"I been telling Ellie she should'a been doing this the whole time she pregnant, but no one listens to some old goat like me. But it's still not too late do it. Even now it's bound to he'p a little."

She had me at "honey spot" and I wanted to hear more. "What do I do?"

"It's easy. Just when that baby of hers is about to be born, you place coupla fingers inside her tiny little vagina and stretch it from side to side. Just like this . . ." The grandmother demonstrated by holding up her two hands, index fingers knuckle to knuckle and extended. Then, keeping her knuckles together, she spread her fingers apart far as they would go.

"You massage and stretch that honey spot with your fingers until that area 'tween her lady vagina and butthole gets soft and thin. You rub like you trying to iron a wrinkle outta a starched white shirt. Before you know it, that honey spot'll open up so wide a grapefruit could pass through with no trouble at all."

I'd heard about the technique before but in less colorful terms. It was called perineal massage. The practice was usually done daily during the last trimester of pregnancy in hopes of lessening chances of tearing during delivery, or the need for an episiotomy. I thought it unlikely to help at this stage of labor, but it wouldn't hurt to give it a try.

Lois spoke up. "What about having Susan stand up against da wall and squat? I seen my grandmother have women do dat many times and it always seemed to help."

She was right. Squatting was another technique used by midwives along with application of fundal pressure during contractions. With fundal pressure, an assistant pushes firmly downward on the uterus during a contraction. The procedure can increase pressure inside the laboring womb and help push the baby out. It can also cause the uterus to rupture and the mother to bleed to death in seconds.

I had determined by vaginal exam that Susan's cervix was completely dilated and she was ready to push out her baby. The obstacles we faced now were her small pelvis with a tight birth canal and a breech presentation.

I couldn't do anything about the small pelvis or the breech, so I decided to try the perineal massage. I had Susan lift her knees again, and with my two index fingers just inside the opening of her vagina, I began a vigorous massage. After just a minute or two, I actually felt her tissue begin to soften and become pliable.

Susan had a firm contraction and with it, I could see a tiny mound of pinkish skin showing through the introitus. The baby had begun its final descent into the birth canal and the perineal massage seemed to be helping open the passageway.

"Now," I said with excitement. "Let's help Susan stand up against a wall and squat."

"You OK to do dat, honey?" Lois asked Susan.

Susan was panting through a firm contraction, but nodded in a way that could only be interpreted as: *Hell yes. Get this over with!*

We helped Susan over to a wall where she stood erect. There, with a woman on each side grasping her by the armpits, we lowered her to a squat.

I placed a towel between Susan's feet then hunkered myself down on the floor facing her. I changed into my second pair of sterile gloves, then readied my arms directly below her pelvis, prepared to make the catch of a lifetime.

Susan moaned with a contraction.

"Now push!" I said to Susan. "Lois, apply firm pressure to the top of her uterus."

Susan held her breath and strained. Her lower body began to shake. Lois pushed.

More pink skin.

"Push again, Susan!" I called out.

Susan took a deep breath, held it firm, and pushed once more.

I spotted two distinct mounds with a crease in between. It was the baby's buttock.

"One more time, Susan. We're almost there!"

"I can't!"

"Of course you can," Lois said and patted Susan on the shoulder. The women in the room chanted louder.

Susan let out her air, sighed and took in another deep breath. She held it and pushed with all the strength she had left in her body.

Then, Susan pushed her baby right out of the birth canal and into my waiting arms, followed by a whoosh of brown-stained amniotic fluid and a flood of bright red blood,.

I turned the squirming infant face down and cradled him in my left arm. I gently patted his back to expel any fluid he may have aspirated that last second before birth and he let out a high-pitched cry.

The remainder of the delivery proceeded without incident. We returned Susan to her cot and I delivered the placenta. I was amazed the perineal massage had prevented a tear in the vagina or rectal wall and no stitches were required. That was a good thing—since I had no suture material with me. We didn't have a cord clip, but one of the attending women pulled a string from a package she'd recently received in the mail, and with it we securely tied off the cord.

We had no way to weigh the baby, but I estimated his weight a minimum of ten pounds. I examined him as best I could; he seemed normal and healthy. The only thing I noticed out of the ordinary was that the child, like his mother, had skin of a slightly lighter tone than other Eskimo babies I'd had the pleasure of delivering since coming to Nome.

We covered the baby in a furry reindeer pelt and I handed him to his mother. Susan smiled and promptly held her newborn to her engorging breasts.

We dodged a bullet with this delivery and I mentally thanked Ellie's grandmother whose advice probably made it possible.

We all smiled and praised Susan for the work she'd done. The elder women in attendance danced and gleefully praised my efforts, treating me with kisses from toothless grins and thanking me for my help. One woman lit up a pipe and offered me a draw, which I respectfully declined.

I wanted to hug all involved, but quickly realized I was soaking wet and covered with bodily fluids that I would be wise to rid myself of as soon as possible.

I checked my wristwatch. It was about eleven thirty in the morning. I found it hard to believe the entire ordeal had taken less than two hours. Now if I could just reach Otis and he could handle the weather, I would be home soon, having lunch with Pat and the kids, and telling all about the exciting adventure I'd had in Golovin earlier in the day.

I thanked everyone for their help and threw my parky over my soiled clothes. I tried to push open the door of Susan's hut. It was stuck.

"Give a little tap with your foot," Lois said.

I did, and the door flew open in a blast of Arctic wind that stung my face like a furnace. I looked out and saw nothing but white. There was no horizon, no sky, no earth.

Lois glanced out the door and shook her head. She helped me pull the door closed.

"April sometimes brings worst storms of da winter," she told me. "Dis one look like might be one of the biggest in years."

It was the last thing I wanted to hear. My clothing was saturated with unmentionable grunge and my face and hair the same. I had no change of clothing, no personal supplies, nothing.

"Can we get to the village radio so I can call Munz Air to come get me?" I asked Lois.

Lois shot me a sad face. "Radio never work in weather like dis," she said. "But don't matter no how. Not even Otis or dat crazy Sparky O'Neil could come get you at da moment. Storm too big. You best get settled in for da night. Could be here in Golovin for quite some time."

CHAPTER 41

I discovered I wasn't cut out for village life.

I spent the first night with Lois Arrluk and her husband, Joseph, bundled up in their tiny hut built of driftwood and tin. They offered me their oldest kid's cot, draped off from the living and cooking area by a plastic shower curtain. I was grateful, of course, but declined out of courtesy. I opted for floor space in front of a makeshift heater that burned seal oil.

Lois's husband, about three sizes larger than me, loaned me some socks, underwear, a pair of jeans, and a flannel shirt. I cinched the jeans up around my waist with a belt made of dried reindeer hide and fur.

My boots were soiled beyond cleaning, so Joseph loaned me a pair of sealskin mukluks, very warm and beautiful. Lois tried cleaning my soiled parky with snow, but the coat was so permeated with odor I questioned whether I'd ever be able to wear it again.

I tried to wash Susan's bodily fluids out of my clothing, but with limited fresh water reserved for drinking, no way to heat it, and no detergent, I eventually gave up, cramming my things into a plastic bag Lois found in her kitchen. I'd take them home and ask Pat to see what she could do with them later.

After the first night of sleeping on a tarpaper floor covered by a reindeer pelt, my back was sore and my legs ached from lack of exercise. Despite the padded comfort of the skin and bulk of the clothes, I couldn't shake the cold that permeated my muscles and bones. Loneliness invaded my mood, vacillating my temperament between frustration and anger.

I needed to find another place to stay. Lois and Joseph shared their one-room home with three children and an oversized husky dog. The last thing they needed was a stranger stuffed in with everyone else.

On the second day in the village I met the BIA teachers, Alice and Franklin Kohls. They were a kind, middle-aged couple from Portland, Oregon, who had taught at the Golovin school over ten years. The Kohls invited me to stay with them in a small apartment annexed to the school. No doubt I would have been comfortable there, sleeping in a real bed, enjoying a real toilet and shower. But early on I had promised myself to never stay with teachers when traveling to villages, believing the bond I could develop with Eskimo residents would be much stronger if I stayed with one of them. It was a promise I now regretted.

"The offer stands if you change your mind," Franklin said. "Just say the word and the room's yours."

I spent one more miserable night on the floor at the Arrluks. Later the next day, the Kohls told me about a small storage room in the school basement that could be quickly outfitted with a cot and lantern. They said I could even sneak up into the main house and use the toilet and shower if I wanted. I wouldn't technically be staying in the main apartment with them and could come and go as I pleased. It sounded like a compromise I could live with, and I accepted.

The third day wasn't too bad. I held clinic in Lois's kitchen for anyone who wanted to brave the whiteout conditions. I had two takers, both kids who had cried all night with earaches. Each ended up with the usual treatment—penicillin shots in the butt every day for ten days in a row! Poor kids!

Lois was keenly aware I wanted to get home. She frequently asked me if I wanted to try the radio, each time footnoting her offer with a comment that no pilot in his right mind would fly in such a storm even if radio contact could be made.

Regardless of Lois's comments, whenever I felt the urge, her husband would fire up the generator so I could give the radio a shot. I tried it several times every day.

"This is Dr. Sims at KMM-426 Golovin calling anyone who will answer. Is anyone the hell out there?" I knew my words didn't follow official radio protocol but fuck it, I wanted to get home. "Does anyone copy me? Mayday . . . Mayday. Does anyone copy?"

I repeated the worthless message so often I literally tired of hearing myself speak. I could only imagine how Lois and Joseph felt.

For the next two days, after repeated tries, I decided to give the radio a rest. I was grateful to Joseph for letting me try, but he was burning his precious fuel every time he started the gen and I certainly did not wish to take advantage of his cordial hospitality or his diesel.

On the fifth day, I removed my wristwatch, thinking the days would go faster if I wasn't constantly checking the time. The storm had worsened and I hadn't seen the sun since I left Nome. Late in the afternoon, during a slight lull in the blizzard, Joseph ventured outside to string a rope between his hut and the schoolhouse. Whenever I wanted to make the trip—to hold clinic, try the radio, anything at all—I was instructed to hold fast to the rope and follow it between the two locations.

I conducted clinic at Lois's hut every morning and tried the radio just once a day. Soon snowdrifts had built up so high around her place that it became difficult to trudge the few yards between her house and my living quarters at the school.

Venturing outside for any purpose was treacherous. I'd been taught in Arctic survival that the best thing to do if caught in a whiteout was to keep moving, so you wouldn't freeze to death, but walk in small circles so you didn't get lost. I heard tales of people being twenty feet away from shelter, but dying because they couldn't see ahead that distance to safety. I figured I was a prime candidate for such demise, so I never ventured out farther than I could see at the end of my arm.

On the evening of my fifth day Franklin, the BIA teacher, brought me a battery-operated transistor radio. He told me KNOM had come back on the air and he thought I might want to hear what was happening at home. I thanked him and set the dial to the familiar 780 AM frequency. I kept the volume low and used its soothing sounds to help me drift off to sleep at night.

It was three in the afternoon on my sixth day in Golovin. The village had been in hibernation the entire week. I had tired of pancakes and Cheerios with dried milk for breakfast and muktuk (whale fat), dried salmon, walrus flippers, seal liver, reindeer meat, and "tundra greens" for dinner. Lunch never happened. Since Lois had no patients and the radio was nothing but static, I decided to spend the remainder of the day in my room catching up on rest. I fell asleep praying the storm would lessen and I'd awaken to a plane landing to take me home.

KNOM was on the air. My buddy Don Pike was playing tunes from the Beatles that lightened my mood. I was half asleep when Don's familiar voice rocked me fully awake:

> "This message goes out to Doc Sims from his wife, Pat," Don announced. "It was recorded this morning in the KNOM studio after she braved the storm to talk with her hubby. Listen up, Doc. This is a good one . . ."
>
> *"Hi, Sweetie. Otis came by and told me he took you to Golovin so I guess you are still there."* Pat's voice sounded soft and comforting but I could tell it balanced on tears. *"We miss you and want you to come home as soon as you can. I wish I could hear from you, just to know everything is OK."* Then her voice began to crack. *"The kids and I are fine and we are all praying for your safety."*

I reached over to increase the radio's volume.

> *"Today is a very special day,"* Pat went on to say. *"Our son got his first tooth and he started to crawl. It was wonderful. I tried to get it on camera but you know I don't know how to work the darn thing. He was just . . .* crackle hiss *. . . and then he . . . almost . . ."*

Dammit! I felt the universe was against me. I grabbed the radio, turned dials, hit it, cussed at it, but all in vain. I could not get the reception back. I wanted to throw the radio against a wall and smash it to bits for betraying me.

But I was certain of one thing I heard Pat say. *Our son got his first tooth and had started to crawl* . . . All I could think was that I wasn't there to be part of it.

I felt an ache in my chest, heavier than I ever thought possible. I decided right then and there, no matter what it took, no matter what I had to do, I would conquer this storm and do anything in my power to get back home.

CHAPTER 42

I passed a restless night, unable to shake the image of my nine-month-old boy rising up on his hands and knees, wavering back and forth with that silly grin planted on his face, courageously trying to make those first crawling moves. I was mad, frustrated, lonely . . . all the emotions that made finding sleep difficult. I wondered about Chantelle, how she was handling her brother's newfound talent and the attention he required from their mother.

I was snoozing when a pounding on my door startled me. I thought it was thunder. Then I heard my name called out.

"Doc Sims. You in dere?" It was Joseph, Lois's husband. He sounded excited. I slipped out of bed, pulled on jeans, and opened the door.

"Where else would I be?" I said to Joseph. He missed my levity and I dismissed it. Something was on his mind.

"Whole village hear bout your boy on radio last night," Joseph said. "We all very sorry you missed what happened."

I shook my head. "Thanks."

"Village elders come up with plan to get you home. You interested?"

That jolted me fully awake. I motioned for Joseph to come in and take a seat. He entered but remained standing.

"Village of White Mountain just across Golovin Bay and up Fish River short ways. Maybe fifteen miles from Golovin over water. We need to get you dere. To White Mountain."

Get me to White Mountain fifteen miles over water? It wasn't possible. Every drop of water between the west coast of Alaska and Siberia was frozen solid.

"White Mountain is only village on peninsula not located right on ocean shoreline. Storms usually not as bad der as here. Elders say if we get you to White Mountain, you have better chance of catching plane back to Nome."

"But the bay is frozen solid," I said to Joseph. "How would I get to White Mountain from here?"

"You leave dat up to me. Just let me know if you want to go and I'll take care of da rest."

It took nothing to make up my mind. *No matter what it takes, I will do anything in my power to get home.*

"Of course I'm interested! When?"

"You be ready to leave by daybreak tomorrow morning."

"OK . . ." I muttered. I would like to have had a little more information than that, but before I could get out another word, Joseph headed for the door. Business concluded.

"Thanks!" I hollered out. "I'll see you in the morning." I held up a hand and gave a feeble wave that wasn't returned. I really needed to get more familiar with stoic Eskimo ways.

DAY 8

I gazed outside to the bleakest weather I had ever seen and shivered. It was unsettling to think that, in just a few minutes, I was going to be right out in its midst. At some point in their lives, everyone wonders how they will die; I found myself pondering the reality that *today might be that day.*

It was precisely six o'clock. I knew that because KNOM hit the air at that hour and I had just heard their signature jingle from the little transistor. Static had somehow cleared during the night.

The outside door of the school building flew open, followed seconds later by a determined knock at my bedroom door. I opened, ready to give Joseph a hearty greeting but much to my surprise, a young Eskimo boy greeted me instead.

"Hi," the boy said in a voice more animated than any I'd yet heard from an Eskimo male. His appearance, like his voice, was atypical as he stood there in a flashy one-piece snowmachine suit and sunglasses. Instead of a fur Eskimo parky, he was decked out in a heavy nylon jacket similar to mine, the one Pat ordered from a mail-order outfit in Seattle she had discovered called Eddie Bauer. The boy's feet and hands were covered, not with mukluks and skin gloves, but with heavy leather boots and snowmachine mittens.

"My name is Peter. They call me Peetie. You ready to head out to White Mountain, my man?"

My man? Did I hear him right? And where is the typical Eskimo accent everyone seems to have? Clearly this kid has not spent all his life in Golovin.

"What's your last name . . . Peetie?"

"Tikaani. It means wolf. Like me." He pounded his chest with both fists and shot me a smile abundant with perfect white teeth.

"Well, come inside Peetie. It's a blizzard out there."

Peetie came through the door, and the way he knocked snow off his boots before entering told me how well he'd been raised. I pulled the door closed behind him.

"So, what can I do for you . . . wolf man?"

"Joseph Arrluk said you wanted to go to White Mountain and I'm taking supplies over there today. You can hitch a ride if you want."

"What kind of a ride? You don't fly a plane, I presume."

"Nah. Not yet anyways," the boy said. "Step outside and I'll show ya."

I threw my parky over my shoulders and stepped out onto the porch. Just outside my door I spotted Peetie's ride.

Pulled atop a snowbank next to the schoolhouse door sat a rusted, scarred Ski-Doo snowmachine connected to an equally tattered wooden dog sled. The sled was loaded top to bottom with stacks of cardboard boxes cinched together with rope. Each stack was about six feet long and eight feet high. A young Eskimo girl, dressed in clothes as equally modern as Peetie's, sat huddled up on the snowmachine seat, clapping her hands to keep them warm.

"Your chariot, my man," Peetie said. He dramatically stretched his arm out, displaying the snowmachine and sled as if he were a salesman trying to make a difficult sale. "Now go grab your gear and let's get goin'."

I thought he was kidding. If I understood him correctly, he was planning to cart me the fifteen miles across the frozen ocean in the middle of this blizzard on this snowmachine? I said I'd do anything to get home, but this was stretching my commitment.

"How old are you, Peetie?"

"How old do you think?"

"Fourteen," I answered.

"Oh, come on, Doc. Gimme a break. I'm seventeen if I'm a day. Old enough to have a hot girlfriend like Bitsy Q over there sharing my sled."

I looked over to Bitsy. She shot me a timid smile and waved.

"And you plan to take me to White Mountain on this snowmachine?"

Peetie thought a second then shook his head. "Well, technically not *on* the snowmachine. More like behind it. On top the boxes."

I wanted to get home more than anything in the world, and I understood getting to White Mountain was the best way to make that happen. But I also wanted to get home in one piece, not as a frozen clump that would one day wash up on some distant Siberian beach when the frozen ocean decided to thaw.

"I can't sit on top of those boxes while you drag this rig over the frozen bay. I'll fall off!"

"No you won't. We'll tie you on."

"YOU'LL TIE ME ON?" That was even crazier. One crash, one slip in the wrong direction and the sled could overturn. Tied on top, I'd be crushed to death.

"Look out over the bay," I said to Peetie. "It's frozen solid and covered in ruts and ice ridges. It would be hard enough to drive around them even if you could see, let alone now when visibility is next to nothing."

Peetie looked out at the landscape and shrugged. "Don't look no worse than every other time I've done it."

"And how often is that?"

"Usually once a week, or whenever they need supplies in White Mountain."

"And what if I fall off the boxes while you're moving? You won't even know I'm gone."

"Sure we will," Peetie said. "That's one reason I bring Bitsy with me today—besides the obvious." He shot me a wink and thumbs-up. "I tie a big rope around Bitsy's waist and give other end to you. You fall off sled, you give hard yank and Bitsy tells me we've lost you."

"Have you ever done this before?" I asked. "I mean, with someone tied on top of your sled?"

"Plenty of times and in weather just as bad. Never with big, important white doctor like you, but don't see how that will make any difference."

I stepped back and looked Peetie up and down. He was very young and loaded with confidence. I wanted to believe him, and I definitely was interested in getting home.

"If you wanna go, Doc, you gotta tell me now. Trip ahead that's gonna take two, maybe three hours. Daylight don't last forever."

"Let me get my medical bag."

Peetie grinned and shook my hand. "Good choice, my man."

CHAPTER 43

I thought, perhaps, I could convince myself the situation *looked* worse than it actually was. Doing so wasn't easy, considering I had a mind reeling with scenarios of all that could go wrong.

"Let me get you an Eskimo sleeping bag," Peetie said. He opened a box and pulled out a long furry sack similar to the one Pat and I used for our snowmachine trips. "It'll keep you warmer than anything you get from the lower forty-eight."

I took the bag and thanked him.

"Now, climb on top the boxes, slip yourself deep inside the fur and pull it up around your face and neck."

Shaking my head in disbelief I did exactly what Peetie wanted. Then Peetie took a yellow nylon rope, tied one end to the base of the sled, and handed the other end up to me.

"Wind that tight across your waist and legs then pass it back to me. I'll tie it on the other side of the sled and cinch you up tight on top the boxes."

"No," I said, and I meant it. It was dangerous enough just being perched on top the boxes as we traveled, let alone being tied directly to them. "I'd rather just hold on. How about tying one end of the rope to the snow-machine instead of the sled and I'll just hold the other end. I'll use it to stabilize myself as we move."

"You're the boss," Peetie said and he did as I asked.

"You can use the rope kinda like reins on a horse when we go over rough areas," Peetie said. "And squeeze your legs and ass muscles together to keep your balance when we go around curves."

Next Peetie tied a second rope, white, around Bitsy's waist, and tossed the other end up to me. "This rope is your lifeline. Never let go of it. If you start to fall, give Bitsy a tug."

I nodded and fashioned a loop at the rope's end for gripping.

Peetie made a few last-minute checks on the boxes then looked up at me and smiled. "OK, Doc. You ready?"

I sighed and gave Peetie a thumbs-up, thinking I was as ready as I ever would be.

Peetie hopped on the snowmachine in front of Bitsy, pulled the starter rope a couple of times, and the old machine roared to life. He turned around and gave me a grin.

"Here we go, my man." I heard him say over the roar of the engine and the whirling of the wind. "Just like ridin' a horse."

I glanced at my watch. We'd been plowing through heaps of snow and ice for less than thirty minutes, yet it seemed like hours. I'd kept my eyes fixed on the two ropes clutched in my hand as they twisted and lobbed in the void between me and the snowmachine. Dropping either one of the ropes could make the difference between life and death.

We hit an icy patch and slid into a spin. The sled twisted and tipped up on its side a solid thirty degrees. I clenched my thighs and buttocks and held fast to the ropes to stabilize my position. We recovered with a hard bump that caused one of the ropes holding the boxes together to split apart. The rope made a sharp snap when it broke, like sound from the throw of a whip. Loosened by the broken rope, the boxes supporting me joggled and one fell off the sled.

I hollered to Peetie that we'd lost a box, but he didn't hear me and kept going.

We hit an ice ridge and the sled tipped up on its side a second time. It bumped, then nearly flipped. Once again, I fought to maintain my position and not fall off.

Dead ahead, I saw an area of open water, black pools of certain death welling up between edges of floating plates of ice. It was my greatest fear. If we rolled and I was thrown into the water, I would either drown in seconds or die of hypothermia before merciful unconsciousness had a chance to settle in.

The boxes continued to slip apart. I dug my heels into the one I sat on, hoping to stabilize myself, but the thickness of the fur bag prevented my boots from gathering purchase. I began to slide and reached out for something to grab. There was nothing except the handrail of the sled and that was behind me and at least three feet below my reach. While I was fumbling around to secure myself, I dropped the lifeline leading to Bitsy's waist.

"Stop!" I yelled to Peetie again. "Stop!"

But Peetie kept going. He and Bitsy couldn't hear me over the roar of the wind and the grunting of the snowmachine engine. Prayer would have been a better use of my voice than hollering.

We hit a rise, like one of those annoying speed bumps in a parking lot. Slamming down, the sled shook so hard my sleeping bag pitched to one side and the boxes shifted. With nothing to grab, my Bitsy lifeline gone, and the boxes no longer bound together, I was at the mercy of gravity. The snowmachine lurched forward as it came down over the rise and the sled followed. The unexpected thrust threw my body backwards and with no forewarning and nothing to grasp, I careened headfirst over the back of the sled and crashed down onto the ice below.

I landed facedown only inches away from open water. Barely able to breathe, I squirmed to rid myself of the bag, like a butterfly freeing itself from a cocoon, and crawled out onto the ice. Stunned by the fall, I waited a moment for my head to clear then stood and looked around.

I was engulfed in darkness and flurries of snow. There was no sign of the snowmachine, no sign of help, nothing to ease my plight. I was lost, prisoner to the elements against which I had no defense. I knew right then I was going to die on this uncharted journey, lost in a storm and frozen to death. Pat would never know what became of me.

Luckily I was dry, but my head hurt and I felt a crick in my neck where it twisted upon hitting the ice. Both arms and legs worked well and without discomfort, so apparently no extremity was fractured.

Far in the distance I heard the drone of the Ski-Doo as it sped away. I frantically waved my hands and cried out, but I knew it was useless. Exhausted from the struggle, I knelt down on the ice and cradled my head in my hands. Already my hands had begun to ache from the cold and my face tingled from freezing wind. All I could do now was wait for the inevitable to happen. I began to sob and hoped the end would come quickly. I remembered reading that freezing was not a comfortable way to die.

CHAPTER 44

I heard a hum, muffled by distance but certainly there. I stood and scanned the horizon but saw nothing. I hollered their names— "Peetie . . . Bitsy . . ."—but I got nothing back in return. I heard the sound again, slightly louder this time but still too far away to determine its source. Maybe it was a voice, or just a turn of the wind. Perhaps it was a mirage, a figment of hope my imagination was granting to ease these last few moments of my life.

Then I heard it again, only this time I was certain it wasn't my imagination. It was the groaning sound of an engine and it was getting closer. I thought I heard my name called out and I lifted my hands to cup my ears.

"Over here!" I hollered against the howling of the wind. "Over here!"

"Doc Sims. . . Doc Sims."

It was Peetie'e voice. Then Bitsy's.

First, I saw the black nose of the snowmachine as it circled around a pillar of ice; smooth and round like the snout of a killer whale spying ice floes for prey. Then a windshield appeared, and peering through it was the face of a determined young Peetie grinning ear to ear. He spotted me and gave a wave.

Peetie edged the snowmachine skillfully around ruts and past the open water until he pulled the Ski-Doo up directly in front of me.

"You OK?" Peetie hollered. "We thought we'd lost you for good."

"I'm OK. Probably a little bruised up, but nothing more."

Peetie rushed over and grabbed me by the shoulders. He spun me around, vigorously brushing snow off my parky to check me over.

"Don't see no blood so I confirm. You're OK," he joked.

I nodded. "How'd you find me?"

"You got Bitsy to thank for that one. She said you been so nervous ever since we left Golovin you been constantly tugging on the rope tied to her waist. Then a few minutes ago, she noticed you weren't tugging anymore and it got her worried. She pulled on your rope and when the end came back to her, she had me stop to check. Easy as shit. We discovered you had fallen off."

I nodded. "After we crossed over that last ridge."

"So it's a good thing you're such a pain in the ass by tugging on rope all the time or we never would've known you were gone."

I laughed, a strange reaction considering moments before I hovered at the brink of death.

"But it's a whiteout," I said. "How'd you track back and find me?"

Peetie tapped his head several times with a gloved finger. "I told you Eskimo boy know what he doing." He gave my shoulder a little punch and grinned. "Plus, it's not snowing hard enough right now to cover over the snowmachine tracks we just left. I just retraced back over them and they brought us here."

"Easy, no?" Bitsy laughed.

I didn't respond.

"My biggest worry was that you might not stay put and try to find us. That's the big mistake people make when lost in whiteout."

I tapped my head, just as Peetie had done. "Thank God white man paid attention in his Arctic survival class."

Peetie agreed. "Now let's get back to it. We should be in White Mountain soon."

"Soon," I said. "It's a whiteout. Which way does your compass say to go?"

"Compass?"

Peetie looked confused.

"You do have a compass?" I asked.

"Nah. I tried using one once but all it did was get me lost."

Dammit, he's messing with me. At least I hoped he is . . .

"Come on, Peetie. Let me see your compass."

Peetie looked me squarely in the eyes then grinned. "Have you forgotten what I said? I'm Eskimo Wolf Man?" The grin widened. Then he spread his arms out like wings of an eagle and howled as if baying at the moon.

CHAPTER 45

I still harbored doubts about Peetie's ability to travel without a compass. As if that wasn't enough, I also I felt his self-confidence was greatly overstated. The trip was taking much longer than he originally said and, contrary to what he promised, I had fallen from the sled and had hurt my back and neck.

Peetie secured me on top of the remaining boxes and we started out. We traveled less than five minutes when the snowmachine unexpectedly sputtered and died. We coasted to a stop and Peetie hopped off to open the engine compartment. He began tinkering inside.

I wondered if the snowmachine had broken down or, God forbid, we'd run out of fuel. Either of those scenarios could be catastrophic.

Peetie fussed around the engine a couple of minutes then lumbered over to me. His lack of swagger told me something was wrong. Panic that tasted like vomit rose in my throat.

"What's happened?" I said.

"Ski-Doo conked out. I think because engine getting too hot. We need to stop and let it cool down."

"How can that be?" I said. "It's freezing outside."

"I had to go slower than usual today and that made it hard for engine to keep cool. Plus, I had to watch for thin ice that might not hold extra weight of sled with heavy doctor on top."

"How's our gas?"

"That running a little low, too. Extra weight plus doubling back to pick you up has used more than I planned for."

"I don't suppose there's some extra gas in one of these boxes?" I asked.

Peetie shook his head. "Sorry, Doc. Never needed it before today."

We had to go slow and we burned extra fuel. We were stranded now, alone and cold and it was all because of me.

Just moments before I felt I was going to die, lost in this godforsaken storm. And now the feeling returned, but this time with a difference. I was still going to die, but unlike before . . . this time I wouldn't be dying alone.

Darkness settled over us, worsened by thick clouds and wind that dropped the temperature to shivering levels. I was hungry and tired. I knew Peetie and Bitsy felt the same.

The kids stayed on the Ski-Doo while I bundled up in the sleeping bag and tried to stay warm. After forty-five minutes, Peetie came to tell me he was going to try firing up the machine. He advised I pray.

I stared as Peetie pulled the starter rope, holding my breath each time he yanked. Once, twice, a third time. The engine coughed and sputtered but didn't catch. Peetie kicked the side of the engine compartment and raised a hand as if giving the snowmachine the finger. Then he pulled off his gloves and, with bare hands clasped together around the handle, heaved the starter rope so hard he slipped on the ice and fell.

"Start you motherfucking piece of white man shit!" Peetie screeched.

That did the trick! The engine burst into life in a billow of black tarry smoke. It was the most beautiful bit of air pollution I had ever seen.

We forged ahead another hour then Peetie brought the Ski-Doo to a stop. He came back to talk with me.

"Gotta check my bearings," he said with an apprehension in his voice I hadn't noticed before.

"How much longer do you think?"

"Don't know. Ask me when I figure out where we are."

I sighed and looked ahead into visibility I estimated was less than twenty yards.

"All I see is ice," I said. "No shoreline."

"Me neither, but don't worry. Land should be on us in a few minutes. At least I hope so, since we don't have enough gas to go much longer."

My eye caught a silhouette on the horizon. At first, I thought it was a shadow cast by a pile of ice ridges, but there were too many peaks for that. When we got closer I could tell that the shadows were trees, large pines, taller and more abundant than any I had seen since arriving in the Arctic. The trees were clumped together in a forest and covered with boughs of snow like flocked Christmas trees. It was unbelievable. We had found a shoreline.

The ice grew thin and cracked as we got closer to landfall making our chances of breaking through higher. Peetie knew it, and crept slowly *around* ice ridges instead of over them and he kept well away from open water. Visibility improved, and soon I spotted a clearing in the trees with a small group of huts huddled together. We inched ahead, and I saw more huts and a white building similar in design to the school we had left behind in Golovin.

The pealing of bells and honking of snowmachine horns welcomed us into the village. As we approached, a band of people came running up to meet us, cheering and waving their arms.

Peetie pulled the Ski-Doo off the ice and without shutting down the engine, leaped off the big machine and ran into the arms of an older Eskimo man. The elder gathered up Peetie in a warm embrace and held him there until I walked up to greet them.

"Doc Sims, I'd like you to meet my father, Robert Tikaani. Dad is Chief Elder of White Mountain."

I reached out to shake the older gentleman's hand.

"My boy good guide?" Mr. Tikaani asked. "It take him many hours to get you here from Golovin today. Whole village starting to get a little worried."

I nodded. "He did a very nice job."

"He quite a boy," the father said, "even dough he not into Eskimo ways as he should be."

"I think he used his Eskimo ways just fine getting us here," I said. "Frankly, I don't know how he did it."

Mr. Tikaani smiled and gave Peetie a hearty smile of approval.

I smiled too and gave Peetie a pat on the back. He had accomplished the impossible. Without the use of a compass or any navigational aids, he had taken us across a hostile frozen landscape filled with hazards and traps and brought us here, safe and alive.

I pulled my parky sleeve up to check my watch. It was just past 6:00 P.M. The proposed two-hour trip had taken over twelve, but it was over. We were now in the comfort of Peetie's home village and all I had to do was look for a way back to Nome.

CHAPTER 46

Lovely people, beautiful scenery, and, of course, a greater chance of getting a plane warranted the risk I'd taken journeying across the frozen sea from Golovin. I was glad I did it, but doubtful I'd ever chance it again.

Joseph was right about the weather in White Mountain. There was less ice and snow, the wind didn't blow a constant gale, and the sky was notably higher than in Golovin. I prayed the better conditions would allow me to get a call out to Munz Northern and they'd send a plane to pick me up.

Opal, the village health aide, greeted me as soon as I said my goodbyes and thanks to Peetie and Bitsy. Eleanor and Bob Faulkner, the BIA teachers, were also quick to make my acquaintance. The teachers sympathized with what I'd been through and graciously offered me a spare bedroom in their schoolhouse apartment. This time I submitted to the temptation, opting more for the comfort of a real mattress and bath than sticking with promises I'd made only to myself. It was an added benefit the village radio was located right in the school, available for my use at any time.

"You look ready to head for your room," Bob said kindly. He pointed towards the schoolhouse and began making his way through packed mounds of snow. I nodded and followed.

The treacherous snowmachine trek had left my twenty-seven-year-old body physically and emotionally drained. I'd been away eight days without a change of clothes, personal items, even a toothbrush or razor and I was weary to the bones. I suffered from a stiff back, sore legs and arms, and a psyche on the verge of collapse. I struggled to contain a sob as Bob lead me to my quarters, explaining away my red eyes and flushed face as the result of freezing wind on the ride over from Golovin. Bob smiled. He understood what I was trying to do. All I wanted now was to find a shower and hit the sack. I could have used a Crown Royal, but no luck in that department. White Mountain was a dry village.

It had never felt better to slip between ordinary bedsheets than it did that night. I slept naked just to feel the smooth texture of cloth and heat of blankets as they caressed my body. The pillow was cuddly soft, a welcomed change from the folded reindeer hide I'd used for the past week, and the covers smelled freshly laundered and clean compared to the skin I'd been using in Golovin.

The room light flickered twice, then went out. The only sound I heard was a clock, hung on the wall of my room, ticking away the seconds until I would find my way home.

DAY 9

At six the next morning, a humming sound caught my attention. The generator hadn't started yet, so the noise was not from that. As far as I could tell, Bob and Eleanor were still asleep, so I doubted the commotion in the house was from them.

The noise grew louder and changed to a deep buzzing tone, like a large insect trying to settle. I realized the sound wasn't coming from inside the house. It was outside. I threw on my jeans and coat and ran to investigate.

Overnight, the sky had changed. Clouds still blanketed the village, but they were weak and transparent. I could even see a glimmer of daylight above the clouds, like sunshine was winning its fight to break away from the heavens and give life back to the earth.

The sound was coming from the south. I spotted its source now, high but descending rapidly and heading straight for me. It was a plane.

CHAPTER 47

The aircraft was still a mile away, but by its rapid descent I believed it was shooting for a landing on the frozen Fish River. Close enough now, I could tell the plane was outfitted with skis, so that was good, but something seemed out of sorts. The plane looked like a Cessna, but misshapen, as if it had been modified in some way. As it got closer I could hear its engine spit and groan like it was under strain and I wondered if the plane was low on fuel or had been weighted down beyond its allowable specs.

The Cessna listed to one side as if having trouble negotiating heavy air. Then, unexpectedly, it plunged and slammed onto the snow-covered river. There was such a bluster of ice and snow I couldn't tell if it landed safely or crashed in a billow of smoke and debris. A crunching, metallic sound filled the air and, once the blowing snow had cleared, I spotted the plane skidding on river ice I feared too thin to support its weight. If that happened, the river would open up and swallow the aircraft and its passengers into a black watery grave.

The ice held and the plane eased to a stop fifty yards upriver from where I stood. I let out the breath I'd unconsciously been holding, relieved I wasn't a firsthand witness to a deadly crash.

The Cessna spun 180 degrees and buzzed toward me. When it got close enough, the reason for its odd appearance and labored flight became evident. Tied onto the plane's skis, one half on each side, lay the gutted carcass of a full-grown moose.

"Sparky O'Neil, you crazy son of a bitch!" I hollered to the bush pilot who was grinning ear-to-ear and waving out an open window of his over-laden plane. "What the hell are you doing?"

"Hey, Doc!" Sparky cried. He cut the engine and hopped out of the pilot seat. He trudged over through piles of snow and threw his arms around my shoulders. "I hear you need a lift to town?"

"You're damn right I do," I said, returning Sparky's hug with a slap on his back. "How'd you know I was in White Mountain?"

"KNOM. Everyone on the peninsula knows you're here and that you've missed your boy's first tooth and crawl."

"I've been trying to reach Munz for days but radio transmission hasn't been working."

"Joseph Arrluk in Golovin kept trying for you after you left. He finally reached someone in Elim who patched a message through to Munz. I've been out hunting a few days, staying inland so the weather wasn't such a bitch, and they radioed me to see if I could get in and get you home."

"With a moose on your skis!" I joked.

"Hey, if you're lucky enough to get a moose there's no way you're not gonna take it home."

I couldn't help but laugh. This was Sparky O'Neil, the most daring Eskimo bush pilot in the Arctic, in his element, doing what he knew best and doing it right.

"So, you wanna a hitch a ride?"

"What do you think?"

"Then grab your shit, say your good-yes, and let's get outta here before we get stuck and I have to share a bunk with you."

I nodded and silently thanked God for sending this crazy, lovable man right when I needed him most.

CHAPTER 48

I stuffed myself into the Cessna's cramped cockpit and buckled in.

"Toss your bag as far towards the rear as you can," Sparky said. "This old bird is gettin' a little lazy and we're gonna need to balance her just right if she's gonna take to the air."

I nodded at the skis. "What about the moose?"

"He's gutted and balanced side to side. It's front to back I'm worried about. With you and me both sitting up here we're gonna be front heavy."

"And that's a problem?"

"Only if you consider flipping head over ass a bitch when we try to take off," Sparky said.

"That doesn't sound good."

"It ain't!" Sparky frowned and shook his head. "It was fine with just me alone up front, but it makes a difference having a heavy doc like you sittin' up here with me."

I wonder if there is any mode of transportation in the Arctic that couldn't kill you at any given moment. And why all this crap about me being heavy? I weigh less now than I did in high school.

"Should I climb in back then?" I asked. "To balance us better."

"God no," Sparky insisted. "I'll need you up here to lunge."

I wondered what the hell *lunge* was. I knew the word but had no idea how it applied to flight. I didn't want to show my ignorance, so I nodded as if I understood and Sparky said no more about it.

"I need to figure out what direction the wind's coming from," Sparky said. "We take off facing it."

"You have instruments to tell you that. Right?" I asked.

"Sure," Sparky said. "This."

Then, in typical O'Neil fashion, Sparky opened up his side window, licked a finger, and stuck his hand outside.

"Ah," he said. "Wind coming from north. That's where I need to point this buggy when I try to get her off the ground."

TRY to get her off the ground? Oh God. After all I've been through, this might be it!

I knew Sparky was crazy nuts and a daredevil, but he was also an accomplished pilot who always came through. He was my ticket out and I decided to trust him.

Sparky gunned the engine and spun us around until he found a position that satisfied him. He flicked a couple of gauges on his flight deck then gazed out the windshield.

"Damn," he muttered. "Just what I was afraid of."

"What?"

"Look ahead of us. The river makes a big curve ahead instead of running straight. You see those trees up there? If we don't get enough speed to give us lift before we hit the curve, we're gonna dump right into that forest."

Blowing snow had cleared just enough so I could see what Sparky was concerned about. The curve with a stand of pines was right in our path of travel.

"OK, then," Sparky said. "No problema . . . "

Oh God, here I go again, trusting my life to an Eskimo man I barely know and whose overabundance of self-confidence could get me into a heap of trouble.

The engine roared, but Sparky kept us from moving. He turned to me with a serious face. "There's only one way we can get enough lift to get us airborne quickly enough," he said. "We have to lunge."

I sighed and wiped my eyes. "All right, goddammit, I admit it. I have no idea what you mean by *lunge.*"

"I didn't think you did, but that's OK. It's easy. When I tell ya, just rock back and forth in your seat, fast as you can. Like this."

Sparky demonstrated what he wanted me to do.

"Cross your arms over your chest and rock like a son of a bitch. Keep your arms high as you can. It'll give us more thrust."

I copied Sparky's actions, but was quickly rebuked for my lack of enthusiasm with the maneuver.

"You look like an old woman in a rocking chair," Sparky grunted. "Roll back and forth on your ass. Do it like there's no tomorrow 'cause if you don't do it right and we hit those trees . . . there won't *be* a tomorrow."

"OK, OK!" I said. I repeated my rocking action, harder and grunting, just like he did. It was more to his satisfaction.

"We call this lunge. Doing this will increase momentum as I try to drag this tug through the deep snow for take-off. I gotta reach at least sixty-five miles an hour."

Oh shit . . . oh shit . . . oh shit.

"Heavy doctor on board make quite the difference in lift," Sparky muttered.

Fuck you about my weight!

Sparky released a brake and the plane lurched forward. "And away we goooo . . ." he hollered.

We jerked and swayed on the icy river surface until the plane found its path. I could feel the skis dragging through the heavy snow as we moved forward and silently prayed as trees and village huts screamed by as we picked up speed.

Just as I felt the plane rumble and a sense of lift in the pit of my stomach, Sparky shouted, "NOW! Lunge!"

Sparky started rocking back and forth as he held tight to the plane's controls. I started rocking the same way.

"Harder," Sparky ordered. "Lean forward and backward more. Rock hard. Pump it. Get your chest all the way to the instrument panel. Get some swing into it!"

I did as instructed. Harder. Faster.

My head began to swim from rocking so fast. We were not airborne yet and the trees were rapidly approaching.

The plane creaked, protesting against the excess weight and strain of the engine.

"Lunge harder, Doc!" Sparky ordered. "We got about another thirty seconds or we're gonna be sittin' on top those bushes."

I lunged so far forward I hit my forehead on the windshield. That's when Sparky let out a belly laugh.

"You can let up now, Doc," Sparky said. "I'm just messing with ya. We got plenty of speed to get lift."

What!

"Yeah," he laughed out loud. "And there's no such thing as lunge. It don't do a damn thing. I got you a good one."

"You shithead!" I hollered. "Look, I bumped by head."

"Oh, poor baby," Sparky laughed. Then his demeanor changed as he turned his whole attention to getting us in the air. He pulled back on the plane's yoke, gave slightly more thrust, and with no hesitation we soared effortlessly into the waiting sky.

CHAPTER 49

A part of me that wanted to knock the bastard out cold for giving me such shit. He had frightened me out of a year's worth of life and I swore, had I known how to fly the damn plane, I would have beaned him one good.

"I'm sorry, Doc, but it was just too good an opportunity to have some fun with ya."

"You made me hit my head," I growled.

"You'll live. Now sit back and enjoy the flight."

I sighed. I had no desire to engage in an argument with Sparky, so I did as he wanted. I leaned my battered head against the coolness of my side window and tried to relax. I closed my eyes and imagined cradling my wife and children in my arms once again. We'd laugh, cry, and give real thanks I was home safely.

We hit a bump and the plane dropped. Fast and hard. I was jarred back into the moment and wondered if Sparky was messing with me again. He wasn't.

"I need to get us above these clouds," Sparky said. "We're still inland, but when I get closer to the coast we'll have rougher air. Our extra weight could be a problem."

That extra weight thing again! Damn.

"Should we set down and drop the moose?" I asked.

"I'd drop *you* before I'd drop the moose," Sparky said. "That's my meat for the next year."

I got it. I didn't like it, but I understood where he was coming from. Meat—even fish by the end of winter—was scarce in the Arctic. If you were able to get some you'd do just about anything to hold onto it.

We hit more turbulence and pitched to the right and downward. The engine whined in protest, the plane shuddered. I felt the muscles in my back tighten.

Sparky adjusted some controls and we settled. My breathing became easier.

"Sparky," I leaned close enough to be certain he could hear me. "Please don't mess with me anymore. I'm not in the mood right now. It's not cool."

Sparky gave me an honest smile. "I'm sorry, Doc. I know what you mean. But don't worry, I will get us home in one piece. I promise to God I will."

The little plane shimmied as we pierced the bottom of the heavy cloud layer. My eyes were glued to the plane's altimeter. It read 1,500 feet.

"How high can this plane go?"

"She's rated at 17,000. I never like goin' much higher than four to five."

"How high will we need to be to clear the clouds?"

"We won't know until we get there. We just keep climbing as high as this tub will go until we break into clear air. We'll need supplemental oxygen if we go above 12,000."

It was more information than I wanted. I figured it best to keep my mouth shut, my eyes closed, and my breathing slow and deep. If oxygen were about to be in short supply, I wanted to take in as much now as I could . . . while the getting was good.

I tried to think of something pleasant. I listened to the purr of the engine and steady whispering of the wind. I could tell we were ascending higher and higher and that felt good. Then something unexpected punched through my eyelids, startling me. Sunshine.

I opened my eyes to blue sky that lay ahead, clean and clear as far as I could see. The altimeter read 9,000 feet as we soared quietly through the open air with heavy clouds below us like a carpet of puff.

"We'll be dropping down into Nome in about ten minutes," Sparky announced. "I've made contact with Nome FAA. We're clear for landing."

It was finally some news I was happy to hear.

"It's gonna be a little bumpy as we drop back into the clouds," Sparky said. "Nothing to worry about. Nome usually has very little wind shear."

I could handle bumpy. It had become the norm. One of the earliest lessons I had learned was that turbulence rarely caused accidents. *Rarely* was acceptable, although I would have preferred *never*. Otis once told me that, historically, there were two fatal crashes every three years between the pilots of Nome and Kotzebue. It was a stat I had little desire to become a part of.

The landing strip was dead ahead. Sparky told me to be certain my seat harness was secure.

I could see there were no planes resting on the tarmac but that was all I could make out. Sparky said he hoped the field had been recently plowed but he couldn't tell from our altitude.

"I'm gonna make a fly over," Sparky said. "I got no report of any problems, but in heavy weather like this no one really checks unless a commercial jet is expected."

"OK," I replied, as if I had any say on what was going to happen in the next five minutes.

"Keep your eyes tight on the runway. Look for any obstacle we might have to dodge as we set down."

"You messing with me now, Sparky?" I asked.

Sparky turned and looked me square in the eyes. He was serious for the first time during the flight. "Not a chance," he said.

We began our descent. The altimeter dropped quickly: 4,000, 3500, 3000, 2000, 1000 feet. We were now close enough to make out details. There was a scattering of vehicles surrounding the airport shack, a truck with an Alaska Airlines logo stenciled on its sides and several snowmachines. We were almost there: 750 feet, 500. It was then that I spotted something which lifted my spirits right out of my seat.

Parked next to the shack, between a snowmachine and a beaten-up pickup, was a yellow Pontiac station wagon. I knew there was only one person who would drive that car out in weather like this to meet our plane. I couldn't wait to take that person into my arms.

Sparky made a perfect touchdown. We taxied up to the shack, and before the engine had completely stopped, I opened the door and shot out of the plane.

"Watch yourself, Doc," Sparky said. "It's a slippery mess out there."

I hobbled my way from the plane to the terminal, but before I got there, the door flew open and there was Pat. We ran into one another's arms like I had just returned from the dead.

"Are you all right?" was all Pat could ask. Several times. "Are you really all right?"

I assured her I was fine. She pulled off her glove and gently caressed the redness on my forehead.

"Does it hurt?" she asked.

"Only when I laugh." I couldn't hold back a grin, and we hugged again.

"Jamie is home with the kids. About an hour ago Billy dropped by to tell me he'd gotten a call from Munz that Sparky had picked you up in White Mountain. We figured you'd be landing about now, so he brought Jamie over to watch the kids so I could meet you. Frank offered to bring me out, but I wanted to come myself."

"Jamie and Billy are the best," I said. "So is Frank. Don't know what we'd do without them."

Pat gently kissed my cheek and forehead then firmly on the lips.

"I don't know what I'd do without them or you," Pat said softly. "And I hope I never have to find out either way."

PART FOUR

THE FINAL MIDNIGHT SUN

"Hope is being able to see there is light
despite all the darkness."
—Desmond Tutu

CHAPTER 50

I 'd heard the migration of seasons from winter to summer would bring changes to village life that might lighten my clinic load. It did not. I yearned for more time with my family but saw no way to make it happen. I had lost weight, I was pale, and I had started to shed my abundance of shoulder-length hair, a trait I considered my most redeeming physical trait.

I had a constant stream of trauma to deal with, babies to deliver, surgeries to perform, every imaginable infectious disease and mental illness to sort out. I dropped routine radio traffic down to five days a week by instructing health aides to restrict weekend calls to emergencies that couldn't wait until the following Monday.

I made repeated pleas to Kotzebue for help, but my requests fell on deaf ears. Why Kotzebue, with everything they had, couldn't be reduced by one or two physicians to join me in Nome was beyond my comprehension.

MID-MAY, 1972. FRIDAY EVENING.

HOURS OF FULL SUNSHINE: ALMOST EIGHTEEN

"You'll hear it first," Ed Greenberg, our local pharmacist, tried to explain. "It's louder than you expect. Then you'll see it. It's called breakup and it's pretty damn neat."

Ed and I were sharing a few beers at the BOT after I'd dropped by his pharmacy to check on some meds I needed at the hospital.

"When does it happen?"

"About this time of year, depending on water and air temperatures. Sea currents I suspect, too."

"And the ice just melts?"

"Hardly," Ed said. He settled back in his chair and spoke up over the blaring music. "The frozen ocean literally blows apart, like someone has set a charge of dynamite. It makes a deafening sound, especially if the wind is blowing offshore. Some years it happens almost overnight. Others, it can take a week or more."

"Rivers at the same time?"

"Usually."

"Then what happens?"

"Once the ice breaks apart, open water appears and everything eventually just flows out to sea."

"So that's it?"

Ed shook his head. "Hardly. The best is still to come. Before the ice makes it out too far, many floes and bergs are still close enough to be reached by boat. They make great hunting grounds for seals."

I paused, taking in everything Ed said.

"Sounds exciting, like something I wouldn't wanna miss."

"Breakup . . . or hunting seals?" Ed asked.

I shrugged. "Both sound pretty interesting."

"Then you should try it."

I took a gulp of beer and wiped my upper lip of foam. "We are talking about watching breakup, right?" I asked.

Ed grinned. "Among other things."

"You mean hunting for seals? On the ice?"

Ed nodded. "Just about everyone does it, getting pelts and seal liver." He made it sound like a rite of passage.

"Are we even allowed to hunt seals? Isn't that something only Eskimos can do?"

"It's the same as fishing and crabbing. It's OK if you have the right license. We aren't allowed to possess walrus ivory except for carvings done by Eskimos and purchased in stores. But we are allowed to catch salmon and hunt seals. Only Eskimos can go after whales and walrus."

I grinned. I really had no interest in whale hunting or capturing a walrus. I'd had more than my lifetime's fill of whale blubber and walrus flippers while weather-bound in Golovin. But the idea of obtaining a spotted seal hide for mukluks was very appealing.

Esther made mukluks from seal pelts she tanned herself and softened by chewing. They sold in stores for $250 a pair. I once told her Pat and I would love a pair and she offered to make us some for just $50 if we could get the skins. I told Ed about Esther's offer.

"She made me a pair a couple of years ago and they cost me plenty more than fifty bucks," Ed said. "That's an offer you can't pass up.

"So, how about it?" Ed said. "You want to set up a little seal hunting expedition when the time arrives?"

I loved to fish but wasn't sure about hunting since I'd never really done it. Ed wanted an answer now, and the brew I'd consumed helped me make my decision. I gritted my teeth and slowly nodded. "Why not?" I answered with as little slur as possible.

We shook hands, and Ed raised his glass in a toast.

"OK, then it's a date," he said. "The first Saturday or Sunday after breakup, let's do it."

TWO WEEKS LATER.
SATURDAY MORNING. EARLY.

I had just gotten home after morning rounds when a rumble echoed through the walls of our trailer. I thought it was an earthquake. Then I realized what was happening.

"Breakup!" I hollered to Pat. "Grab the kids!"

We threw on our boots and coats and Pat pulled a blanket around the children. The trailer was just two blocks away from shore and we didn't want to hassle with the car or snowmachine.

"Let's run," I said.

In less than five minutes, we were standing on the boardwalk, staring out at the Bering Sea and the remarkable event unfolding before our eyes.

❖

It was just as Ed foretold, only far more spectacular than I imagined. First, huge cracks spread across the surface of the frozen sea, dissecting in zigzag patterns as they traveled to and fro. A screeching electric sound filled the air like the cries of a thousand seagulls. The sea's frozen surface succumbed to the cracks and swiftly tore to pieces, creating mountains of ice that crashed down into the waiting ocean. The icy mountains sank at first from their mammoth weight, then found their buoyancy and bolstered upwards toward the sky like rockets. The mountaintops hovered, suspended for a moment as they reached their summit, then with a thunderous roar avalanched back down into the sea as icebergs and floes. The ice mountains heaved and sank in the cobalt water, repeatedly, in a slow-motion dance until they found their perfect balance. Pulsations from their rise and fall gave birth to sun-capped breakers that blustered onto the shoreline of Nome in sparkling, foamy crests.

The spectacle lasted over two hours, then gradually the sea quieted. As its surface calmed, lakes of still, open water rose up between the edges of the floes and, like a natural mirror, reflected in perfect harmony every soft wispy cloud that hovered above in the Arctic sky.

CHAPTER 51

You ready?"
    I opened our front door and laughed at Ed Greenberg, standing there as the image of Davy Crockett with his parka zipped up to his five o'clock shadow and a rifle hoisted over his shoulder. He wore a grin on his face that wouldn't quit. All he needed was a coonskin cap and the resemblance would have been complete.

I invited Ed in for a cup of coffee, but he declined. "No time," he muttered. "We gotta bust outta here before the ice heads over to Siberia. Gather up your gear and let's go."

The evening before, I had asked Billy if I could borrow his .22 rifle. He was happy to give me the gun and included a box of shells. He told me to watch myself and not shoot myself in the foot or anyplace else that might cause me grief. We laughed and then I headed home to hit the sack. Ed said he'd pick me up early.

"You want a lunch?" Pat asked as I was heading out the door. Ed was within earshot and answered for me.

"We be real Alaska seal hunters, madam. Have beer for lunch. Maybe whiskey. No need for other food and I've got that booze thing covered."

Pat grinned and shrugged. "OK, big guy," she said. "Now you take care of my man. He's new to this kinda thing so go easy on him."

Ed's seventeen-foot aluminum skiff was on a trailer attached to his pickup. I hopped on board the truck and twenty minutes later, we were rounding the Nome jetty preparing to launch the boat into the Bering Sea. We loaded our gear into the skiff, got the boat settled into the water, and I hung a set of heavy camouflage-painted binoculars around my neck. I scooted myself up to the first of three aluminum slat benches inside the boat and took my seat.

The sea was calm, and the boat held steady. Icebergs were everywhere, white blocks in strange forms and shapes that glistened in the rising morning sun. Some were no larger than a car. Others were huge like floating mountains. All were surrounded by rugged edges and sharp peaks, and all floated in the bluest water I'd ever seen.

"Keep looking for flat areas on the bergs, especially next to the water's edge," Ed said. "That's where the seals are. I'm gonna keep the motor just above an idle so I won't scare anything off."

I nodded.

"We may come across a walrus or two. Shouldn't be any problem unless it's a big bull that's hot for a mate. In that case, we may have to hustle away."

Great. I'm gonna be killed by a horny walrus on the Bering Sea. That should make an interesting epitaph.

"So what do I do if I spot a walrus and he's not happy we're around?"

"Try not to shit your pants. They can be mean."

"OK," I said reluctantly, thinking perhaps I could live without spotted seal mukluks after all. If I mentioned my reservations to Ed, I would never live down the shame. So I stuck with the plan, all the while wondering if an angry, sex-starved walrus was capable of sinking a seventeen-foot aluminum boat with two white guys on board.

"Look for a seal with light-colored fur and black spots. They make the best-looking boots. Look for an adult, not a pup. Spotted seals are smaller than other black or brown seals. Sometimes it's hard to tell the difference."

As we floated quietly through the garden of icebergs, many thoughts drifted through my mind. One realization, very unpleasant, was that we were out hunting seals and soon I would be expected to make a kill. Sure, I would use the hide for mukluks, eat the liver, and give the rest of the meat to Esther. The kill was justified, but I didn't like the idea of taking the life of another living creature. The thought weighed heavily on me.

Something splashed in the water straight ahead. I prayed it wasn't a walrus with a hard-on for our boat. Then I heard a hacking sound, not unlike a dog with a case of kennel cough. I lifted the binoculars up to my eyes, scanned, and saw nothing. I heard the sound again. It was coming from around the corner of a large iceberg that floated directly ahead.

"Hold up a second," I whispered to Ed.

He cut the engine and we drifted silently.

I heard it again, three barks, all of the same timbre. Then quiet.

It had to be a seal. Maybe the kind we were searching for.

Ed used an oar to move the boat without a sound. Just as we were about to round the corner of a large berg, I spotted a fully-grown, beautifully marked spotted seal. It had silver-white fur sprinkled with a mixture of black and brown spots over its entire body. I couldn't tell its sex, but prayed it wasn't a female with pup. I wanted it. I felt certain it would make a fine pair of mukluks.

The seal was lying right next to the water's edge as if sleeping. Our boat caught a small wave and we bumped the ice. The impact startled the seal and it raised its head to look around.

"Oh my God," Ed said. "That's the one." He said the words louder than he should have. "You'll never find a better. Take your shot quickly."

The seal reacted to Ed's voice, turned its head and stared right at me. Its beautiful almond eyes sparkled in the morning sun and we were so close I swore I could sense the warmth of its breath. It pulled itself up on its front flippers as if standing at attention.

I raised the gun and squinted through the sights.

"Shoot, Tom. Now!" Ed hissed.

I took careful aim at the seal's head, wanting to avoid a bullet hole through the pelt of the neck or chest. The seal held its gaze on me, as if knowing what I was about to do.

I didn't move. I didn't even breathe.

"What are you waiting for, dammit!" Ed said again. "Shoot!"

I felt severe pressure to yield to Ed's demands to kill the seal. I had told him I wanted mukluks and had asked him to take me hunting so I could get a pelt. Now I regretted those words.

"This is what you came for, Tom. Take the shot!"

Ed's demands burned through my head. *Take the shot . . . take the shot.*

I raised the rifle to position and took one last peek through the gun's sights. I sighed, then squeezed my eyes tightly shut and pulled the trigger.

The snapping sound of the gun jolted my eyes wide open. The seal flinched, so I knew I'd hit it.

"Shoot again," Ed said. "You connected but he's not down. Esther can cover over any bullet holes."

The seal grunted, then arched its back and began scooting towards the water. It stopped, turned its head and stared back at me. I raised my gun, took second aim, but hesitated. I just couldn't do it.

"Goddammit, it's getting away. SHOOT!" Ed shouted.

I lowered the gun and peered into the seal's eyes, noticing how sad they looked. It was as if he was wondering why I would want to harm him. I actually felt as if I'd made a connection with the creature and, at that very moment, knew I'd made the right choice to not fire again. The seal turned its head away from my gaze and arched its beautiful body. I held my breath as it slowly slipped off the ice and into the depths of the surrounding sea.

"Shit!" Ed said. He started the boat's motor and raced over to the area where the seal first lay.

"Check the water!" Ed shouted. "See if you can find it floating."

I searched around the sloshing water churned up by the boat's motor, but saw no sign of the seal. I prayed I wouldn't. I scanned the edge of the ice, saw drops of blood confirming I'd hit the animal, and felt my stomach surge.

"Do you think I injured it badly?" I asked Ed, hoping for a response I could live with. Ed gunned the boat, cussed and swirled us around, examining the water for signs of the injured animal.

"Impossible to tell, but there's not much blood. If doesn't break the surface in a few minutes we can pretty well assume you didn't hit it anyplace critical and it probably just swam away."

I found myself hoping against hope that was what happened.

"Why didn't you shoot again? I'm sure you could have gotten it down before it took to the water."

"I guess I'm just not much of a hunter," I answered. "Sorry."

"Don't apologize to me. I'm fine. You're the one not getting the mukluks."

I shrugged. "Yeah, I guess you're right." I took a deep breath, tried to clear my head. "I'll survive."

"You wanna keep trying for another one?" Ed asked with a tone that was clearly frustrated. I was sorry for that, but not as sorry as I would have been had I killed that sweet, innocent animal.

"You know what, I don't think so. I'm pretty upset with myself for missing the shot and not taking another. I can't honestly say what came over me."

I lied, but don't think it fooled Ed. He simply smiled, shrugged a shoulder and put his gun away. He turned the skiff around and we headed back toward shore.

Just as we were entering the jetty, Ed turned to me. "You know, not everyone can be as heartless as me. I'd have done whatever it took to bag that seal." He paused. "But that's just me."

"You're home earlier than I expected," Pat said as I walked through the door. I explained the whole ordeal and hoped a long philosophical discussion wouldn't ensue. It didn't. Instead, Pat made very light of the story and asked me if I wanted something to eat. I'm sure she felt that giving me time to process what happened would be the best way for me to handle it. As usual, she was right.

I was upset for days after the seal hunt. I felt no malice against Ed and his love of the hunt. It was fine for him. Shooting the seal for boots and meat was not wrong. The error in judgment came when I thought *I* could shoot the seal. *Killing betrayed my nature.*

That day I came to realize the enormous influence peer pressure has over actions. I took the first shot because I felt pressured and therefore succumbed to what I believed my friend *wanted* me to do. I did it rather than remaining strong of spirit, sticking with what my heart told me was right.

I vowed to myself that would never happen again. When faced with difficult decisions in the future, I would tally up my intellect and emotions and allow my heart equal influence with my head before deciding how to act. I learned that, more than likely, whichever way my heart leaned was probably the way I should proceed.

CHAPTER 52

T he exorbitant cost of food, fuel, arctic clothing, and yes, our occasional
visit to the BOT and Friday night buffet at the Golden Nugget,
soon depleted everything we had in checking and savings. We were barely
making ends meet with my PHS salary come the end of every month. It
wasn't that we were overspending; we were undercompensated.

The message was clear. I had to earn more money.

I hadn't been home from the hospital five minutes when I heard a knock
at our front door. I'd been up most of the night with one emergency after
another and was ready to spit nails when Pat answered to a man dressed
in a business coat and tie; a most unusual attire for Nome. It was enough
to stir my interest.

The man introduced himself as Peter Jackson and said he represented
an insurance company out of Anchorage. Oh God, I thought, even here
in the Arctic door-to-door salesmen can be found.

Jackson asked for a few minutes of our time and against my better judge-
ment, Pat invited him in and offered coffee. After a minute of small talk,
he got down to the reason for his visit.

"Every few months I come to Nome to see potential new clients," Peter explained. "I usually have about ten new enrollees every time."

I yawned, suspecting next would be the sales pitch he'd come to deliver. I figured it would be about life insurance, a subject that couldn't be further from my mind. I was just about to cut our visit short, fibbing that I needed to get to the hospital, when he got to the real reason for his call.

"Every one of my new clients will need a physical exam and I was wondering if you'd be interested in doing those for me. The pay would be $25 each and you could do them in the evenings, right here in your own home."

I felt like I needed to have him repeat himself, as if I hadn't heard him right. Peter didn't look like an angel, but his message was a voice from heaven. Less than a year before I was willing to go days without sufficient sleep yet still moonlight at the San Joaquin General emergency room for $8 an hour. Now this man was offering me the equivalent of three times that amount for a simple exam I could do right in my own living room.

I didn't need to ask Pat what she thought about the offer. Peter and I worked out the details and he said I'd have my first case in just a few days.

After Peter left and Pat and I had settled our excitement over the good fortune, I took to my favorite chair for a little snooze. I had just drifted off when came another knock at our front door. This time, standing on the porch, with a terrified look on his face, was a middle-aged Eskimo man clutching a blood-soaked animal to his chest.

"Doc, it's my husky Nuk. He got bad cut on head and neck."

"Come in," I said. I hollered for Pat to make a place on our kitchen table. "What's your name, sir?"

"Herald Kowlaka," the man answered.

Herald rushed in and laid his dog on the table. I unwrapped a blanket thrown around the pet and dug through dirt and dried blood in search of the wound. When I found it, I was taken aback by the severity of the injury.

A deep, filthy, eight-inch gap encircled the dog's neck like he'd been hung from gallows. An array of muscles, tendons, blood vessels and a nodular tube I recognized as his trachea protruded through the jagged edges of the massive wound.

"What happened?" I asked Herald.

"It's all my fault. I chained Nuk up to back of pickup but forgot he was der." The man began to weep. I'd never seen an Eskimo male do that. "I drove off with him still attached and dragged him at least quarter o' mile before I realized what I done."

I'd heard such a tale before but considered it an urban legend. Now, it wrenched my gut to see it could really happen.

Nuk was unconscious. His labored breathing was accompanied by gurgling sounds made by air rushing out through a tear in his windpipe. And he was wheezing, an indication his airway was obstructed. I knew if I didn't quickly clear the obstruction in his trachea and close up the tear, Nuk would suffocate in a matter of minutes.

"Steady his head," I told Herald.

I pried Nuk's mouth open and sunk in a finger deep inside his throat. I rummaged around until my finger hooked something. I pulled it out and his wheezing improved. What I removed was half his tongue.

Dark red blood spurted from lacerated arteries and veins deep within the dog's neck. Skin from the left side of his muzzle had been sheared away leaving only a bloody mass of muscle, bone, and teeth in place. Much of his upper lip, cheek, and lower eyelid on that side had been ripped open and an eyeball was left dangling from its socket by the optic nerve.

I looked at Herald and frowned. It didn't take words for him to understand how serious I thought his dog's condition was.

I needed help and asked Pat if she was up to the challenge. The kids were napping, and she finally had some time to herself. But graciously she nodded, her eyes saying she would be happy to do all she could.

We had no way to tell if Nuk had suffered brain or internal injuries, so all we could do was patch up his wounds and wait. I explained the gravity of the situation to Herald and he told me how his kids had grown up with the dog and how he'd never find proper words to tell them what he'd done if the dog didn't survive.

In human trauma, once a victim's vital signs have been stabilized and their bleeding controlled, the first step is cleaning and debriding to avoid infection. I figured the same would apply to dogs. Pat prepared a dishpan full of soapy water and we vigorously scrubbed all wounds of clotted blood, roadway debris, and denuded tissue. Nuk began to move, so I gave him a shot of Thorazine—a potent antipsychotic sedative I kept in my medical go-bag for psychiatric emergencies. Once the sedative took effect, I infiltrated all the injured areas with local anesthetic and we went to work.

First, we repaired the tear in Nuk's windpipe with 4-0 Chromic absorbable suture. We used a turkey baster to provide irrigation and suction. His breathing immediately improved.

Next, we addressed the wounds on Nuk's face. I returned the eyeball to its socket and anchored it in place with stitches. I used a piece of skin to create a new lower eyelid and even though I had no hope the eye would ever see again, I felt the dog would look better with two eyes instead of one.

For the next three hours, Pat and I cleaned wounds, cut away worthless pieces of muscles and fat, and sutured together tissue we thought had a chance of healing. By the time the Thorazine and local anesthetic had worn off, we'd done all we could.

Nuk tried to stand. He was groggy from the sedative shot, but he seemed in very little distress considering what he'd suffered. He coughed several times, sputtering frothy slime from his mouth and nose, which I reassured Herald was a natural reaction to clearing his lungs. I told Herald once Nuk was fully awake he could take him home.

"Keep him in the house, warm, and watch over him. Come get me if you think there's a problem."

Herald wiped his eyes and started to reach down to gather up his dog. Then he stopped and turned to face me.

"I don't know how to t'ank you, Doc," Herald said. He reached in a pocket and removed two twenty-dollar bills that he handed to me.

"This ain't much but it's all I have right now. I get paid from the NC next week and I'll bring you more."

I shook my head. "That's not necessary, Herald," I knew how hard he worked for his money and was more than happy to have helped him.

"Yeah it is, Doc, even if Nuk doesn't make it. You and the missus did all you could and dat's really worth a lot."

Herald held firm on his intent to pay and so I accepted the money as he insisted.

❖

Thus began my unofficial veterinary practice in Nome and my insurance physical moonlighting job. I worked a great deal at both. I never charged locals for vet services more than they could afford and often did the work for free just to insert myself as part of the community.

The extra income I did earn from the new endeavors enabled us to weather the storm of our financial issues. We placed our order for next year's food supply and had some left over for a little R and R.

CHAPTER 53

"A goal without a plan is just a wish."
—Antoine de Saint-Exupéry

As winter temps warmed and sunlight flooded the Nome landscape, patches of spongy emerald tundra grew up from the land and flourished. The greenery, tucked amongst mounds of wind-sculpted snowdrifts left scattered across the treeless plains after the thaw, replaced the barren dead of winter and allowed the Arctic to, once again, spring to life. Icy patches along the roadways melted under heat from passing vehicles and as I walked along those roadways, my spirit was lifted when I noticed that in an inch of puddle I could see a mile of sky.

Villagers enjoyed the springtime thaw and increased daylight as much as I did. Travel between villages became easier and along with travel came the rekindling of a gossip phenomenon known as the Tundra Telegraph. Although huge in size, the Arctic, in many ways, worked like a small town, fueled by legends and stories, none more intriguing than the saga of Piccolo Pete.

Peter Stiles lived a hard life. As a skinny little white man with a freckled face, flaming red hair, and scraggly beard, he was known around Nome as Piccolo Pete because of whistling sounds he made when he spoke. Pete had suffered numerous fractures to his nose and sinuses while trying to negotiate life's troubled years, injuries which had caused changes in his voice to become permanent. He hated the nickname he'd been saddled with, but learned to accept it after bearing its affliction for over forty years.

Pete lived on the edge of town in a shack built of tin and tarpaper, and on the edge of life suffering from extreme hypochondriasis and paranoid schizophrenia. I saw him frequently in clinic because of his cancer phobia. I knew Pete's psychiatric history from reading his medical charts and, although he always struck me as more than eccentric, I always considered him completely harmless.

EARLY JUNE, 1972

I preferred my clinic window open so I could smell the sweet scent of summer tundra. One midafternoon, I heard the whine of a small plane's engine flutter as it approached the Nome airport. I'd come to recognize the familiar drone of this particular aircraft. It was the Alaska State Trooper plane, and it only came to Nome when something was amiss.

"I need to see Doc Sims right now," Alaska State Trooper Darryl Sorenson barked in the rugged, commanding voice he was well known for. "Go get him."

I was in an exam room with a patient but could clearly hear Darryl's voice through the door.

"He's with a patient," Esther told him, unintimidated by his tone. "You'll have to wait your turn. Like everyone else."

"I'm not sick, Esther, it's official business. Go get him."

I'd seen Darryl in clinic a couple of times for minor illnesses and knew he was sincere in performing his job. I figured whatever he needed was genuine, so I excused myself from my patient and went into the hallway to see him.

"Hello, Darryl," I said. "What can I do for you?"

"You know Peter Stiles?"

"Piccolo Pete?"

Darryl nodded.

"Everyone in town knows him. What's up?"

"We all know he's a little light in the squash, but this time he's gone too far. The damn son of a bitch is sittin' on top a hill outside White Mountain with his rifle, taking shots at people floating down the river."

"Jeez."

"Thank God he hasn't hit anyone yet, but it's just a matter of time until he does. Then he'll be wanted for murder."

"Has he done anything like this before?" I asked.

"Never. He has a record of disturbing the peace, public drunkenness, but never anything violent. Have you seen him here in the clinic before?"

I nodded. "He's a bit of a hypochondriac. Comes in often, usually with minor complaints. He's worried he has cancer."

I asked Esther to bring me Peter's medical file and I quickly glanced it over.

"Does he have cancer?" Darryl asked.

"Not that I'm aware of. He has a lot of allergies and facial fractures. He's been hospitalized in Anchorage three or four times for mental disorders. He hears voices and is deathly afraid of the police—thinks they're out to get him."

"We've met with him on occasion."

"I've heard he keeps mostly to himself and only comes into town when he needs supplies. Lives out by the cemetery, I think."

"Yeah, we know that," Darryl said. "We had the Nome police check out his place. It's a filthy wreck. Beer cans and booze bottles slung all over the place. Hardly any food. There's a skinned seal hanging over a barrel to collect the fat drippings for heating oil. They found a couple of empty boxes of 30-30 rifle shells thrown on the floor. We checked with Munz Air and they flew him out to White Mountain yesterday on a one-way fare."

"That doesn't sound good."

"No, it doesn't. A village elder of White Mountain, Robert Tikaani, got a radio message to the state trooper office in Anchorage this morning. Told them about what Pete's doing. He said men in the village were going to gun him down before he kills someone. We asked him to wait until we got there."

"I know Robert. Did he agree?"

"He gave us four hours. That was over an hour ago."

I slipped off my white clinic coat and sat down. "So, what's your plan?"

"We're heading out to White Mountain right now. I stopped by to get you 'cause you're coming with us."

"Me . . . no. Jesus—what do you expect me to . . . ?"

"Look, Doc, we all know Pete is a head case, but it would be a real shame if we had to shoot him. I figured you'd be able to think of a way to take him down without him getting killed."

I shook my head. "You're wrong, Darryl. This is way outta my league. I have no idea what I could do to help you."

"Doc, I grew up in White Mountain and have family and friends there. So I'm not asking you to help, I'm telling you. You better start working on a plan quick 'cause when that plane leaves in the next ten minutes, you are going to be on board."

"For Christ's sake, Darryl."

"It's that or I'm arresting you for obstruction."

"Are you kidding me?" I spit the words out.

I could see the intent in Darryl's eyes and knew I had no choice but to comply with his wishes.

"Can I get a message to my wife to let her know I'm leaving?" My heart was pounding so hard I had trouble catching a breath.

Darryl shook his head. "No time." He hollered to Esther. "Get someone over to Doc Sims' trailer to let his wife know I'm taking him out to White Mountain on an emergency. Tell her we don't know how long we'll be gone."

"Ok," I grunted. I reached behind the door and snapped up my medical bag.

"You all set?" Darryl asked.

"Not in the least!"

CHAPTER 54

Sparky O'Neil was our pilot for the day. He said our thirty-minute flight to White Mountain was going to be a white-knuckle roller coaster ride—something we in the bush referred to as a "Sphincter Level 3." We'd be flying over water, and he warned that heavy summer down drafts, powered by solar winds from the North Pole, could stir the air over the colder Norton Sound waters so intensely the winds could whip a small aircraft like ours through the clouds like an oak leaf caught in a gale. Without any warning, a small aircraft could plummet several hundred feet then spin and crash into the harsh waters of the Norton Sound below.

We shook and shimmied across the clouds and Sparky held the plane the best he could. Periodically he would glance over my way and shoot me a grin that implied the look on his face would be the last thing I would ever see before I met my death in the depths of the Bering Sea.

He was a crazy guy, but Sparky knew his job and got us on the ground in White Mountain without incident. We rolled to a stop and as I was climbing out of the Cessna I noticed a band of people approaching on

ATVs. I counted four men; each dressed in jeans and sweatshirts. They parked their ATVs close to our plane and walked up to us.

"Hello, Uncle." Darryl said.

The oldest of the men nodded. "Haven't seen you in long time, Darryl. Hope you are well."

"I am, Uncle. I understand you've met Doc Sims from Nome. He's here to help us."

I extended my hand. "Hello, Mr. Tikaani. It's nice to see you again. I only wish it was under better circumstances."

"When did you and Doc Sims meet?" Darryl asked his uncle.

"When he was weather-bound here in White Mountain last winter," Robert said. "He make me new glasses when he here."

We all laughed, then the conversation turned to the issue at hand.

"How you plan to get Piccolo Pete off mountain now that you a big state trooper man?" Robert asked Darryl.

"Hopefully without violence."

"You not answer question. How you plan to do dat?"

Darryl turned and nodded towards me. "That's why we brought Doc Sims. He's going to advise us what to do."

"May I say something?" I asked.

Darryl nodded, and I turned to face Robert.

"I know how serious this situation is and I promise to do everything I can. I know some things about Pete that may help us. I only ask you allow me a chance to see what I can do before extreme measures are taken."

Robert turned to Darryl. "What you think?"

"I think we should give Doc a chance. If he doesn't succeed," Darryl tapped the gun on his hip and raised his rifle, "I'll take over."

"OK," Robert said. "But you better make good, Doc. Many lives depend on you."

I had a plan and prayed it would work. If it didn't, someone was going to die today.

CHAPTER 55

Where exactly can I find Pete?" I asked Robert Tikaani.

The elder pointed to a hill on the opposite side of the landing field. "About two miles from here."

"Can you get me close with your ATV?"

Robert nodded.

"Then I'd like you to take me there, but not so close Pete can hear us coming. And Darryl, you need to come separately and stay out of sight."

"Wait a minute," Darryl spoke up. "I can't let you go up there alone. It's way too dangerous."

"We don't have a choice. Pete knows me and he sure as hell will recognize your uniform. If he sees you the ball game's over."

Darryl's eyes told me he got my point.

Pete is a paranoid schizophrenic. He's afraid of the police. Thinks they're out to get him.

"So what are you going to do . . . hypnotize him?" Darryl asked.

"Something better. I have an idea that might allow you to take him peacefully without anyone getting hurt. He needed me once at the clinic and I helped him. He trusted me then and I think he'll trust me now."

❖

It took over twenty minutes to motor up to the ridge where Piccolo Pete sat with a rifle on his lap. Once there, we parked the ATVs behind a rise and I asked Robert and Darryl to remain out of sight until I called for them or they heard a gunshot. Both agreed.

"Which way?" I asked Robert.

"Hike to top of hill. There you will see a path Eskimo hunters use during caribou season. Follow path as it heads down towards river. You'll see Pete."

Robert kissed his fingertips then waved them to the clouds, muttering something I guessed must have been an ancient Eskimo prayer. Then he gave me a thumbs-up that promptly morphed to a fist pump. He followed that with a smile that stretched across his old wrinkled face as wide as the valley below.

CHAPTER 56

The hike up the steep rise packing my twenty-five-pound medical bag over my shoulder winded me, yet I felt surprisingly calm considering what I might be walking into. In the next few minutes I would be staring into the barrel of a 30-30 rifle, pointed by a demented man whose very intent was to shoot me if he felt threatened. I had nothing to protect myself with, save my medical bag and my ability to think.

I found Pete sitting right where Robert Tikaani said he would be, hunched over, hand on his chin, rifle cradled in his lap. His unblinking eyes stared at the river as if mesmerized by the water's movement. Even from my distance I could hear the whistling of his respirations as he anxiously awaited his next target.

Pete wore ragged boots and even more ragged pants and coat. His head was covered with a torn red stocking cap that contrasted harshly with the grayish-red dullness of hair that protruded from around its edges.

I approached slowly and rustled my boots hoping he would hear me coming and not be startled.

"Hello, Pete," I hollered, praying he wouldn't shoot first and ask questions later. "It's Doc Sims, from Nome."

Pete leapt to his feet and spun around. He drew the rifle up to firing position and squinted narrow eyes over the firing sight. The whistling respirations stopped as he held his breath to take aim.

"Click . . . click . . . bam . . . bam . . . Now you'll be a dying man." Pete wheezed.

"No! Pete, hold on there! It's me, Doc Sims."

Pete lowered the rifle and wiped his eyes. He squinted in the bright sunlight.

"Doc Sims?" he shouted.

"Yeah."

"Well, what in the hell are you doing out here?"

I took a step toward Pete. I was relieved that his whistled breathing had started back up, indicating he was no longer in panic mode.

"I was in the village holding clinic and wanted to go for a little walk before heading back to Nome. Surprised to see you here."

"Hmmm . . ." Pete muttered. "Well hell's bells, I think that's a load of bullshit." He raised the rifle to firing position again.

"Pete, how 'bout putting that rifle down," I said slowly. "I just want to say hello."

Pete hesitated. "OK, hello. You said it, now scram." Then he lowered the gun and sat back down on the rock to resume staring at the river.

I joined him on the rock and slipped off my jacket so the Arctic sun could warm the chill inching down my spine.

"Pete, I've been trying to talk with you but haven't been able to find you."

Pete turned to face me. "I've been busy."

"Remember that last time I saw you in the clinic and I did those blood tests for cancer?"

"I remember."

"Well, the lab in Anchorage did some more tests on your blood and came up with something of concern we need to discuss." The lie flowed from my mouth like syrup and Pete leaned closer. His breath nearly gagged me.

"That was a goddamn month ago," Pete grunted. "You told me everything was OK!"

"I know I did, but that was before the lab did additional tests."

"You fucked up, you mean! I knew it! I knew I had cancer. Goddamn you!" Pete began to shake and drew the rifle up to his chest.

"No, Pete. I didn't make a mistake. Put the rifle down. I just got the information yesterday. I think we should go back to Nome so I can do some more tests."

"I should just fucking shoot you dead!" Pete screeched. He bolted upright, stomped his feet on the ground and fired a shot into the air.

"Pete, calm down! I'm here to help you."

"Go fuck yourself!" Pete cried, then dropped down to the ground and buried his head in the tundra. He began to sob. Over his shoulder, I saw Robert and Darryl running toward us. Darryl had his rifle pointed directly at Pete.

Dammit! I was getting somewhere, but if Robert or Darryl showed up, all would be lost.

Pete didn't see Robert and Darryl coming so I took a chance. Hoping he wouldn't notice, I waved my arms, motioning for Robert and Darryl to back away and stay hidden. They understood and slid back behind the rise.

I wanted to comfort Pete so I put my arm around his shoulder, but he pulled away.

"Leave me alone!" he commanded. "Touch me again and I'll kill ya."

The wind had come up, and I pulled my jacket back over my back and chest.

"Pete, let me take you back to Nome today for some more testing."

After a moment, Pete looked up. "Now I know why I was supposed to come to White Mountain. The people here gave me cancer. I need to punish them and then I'll come to Nome."

"Pete, that's not true. People in White Mountain didn't give you cancer. Why would you think that kind of thing?"

"They fed me moose. It tasted funny 'cause it was doused with cancer-causing chemicals."

"That's not true, Peter. I'm a doctor. I know about these kinds of things."

"It is true, goddammit!" Pete spat, he rolled over and fired another shot into the air. "It's their fault, and the whole fucking village is going to pay the price."

Clearly Plan A isn't going to work. I need to move on to Plan B.

My second idea was weak, edgy, and subject to failure. To succeed I would need to lie to Pete again, betray his trust, and call upon his paranoid tendencies and hypochondriasis. The thought made my stomach turn because, if it didn't work, I'd be forced to call in the troops and Pete would likely go home in a body bag.

"How long have you been up here on the ridge, Pete?" I asked. "It's cold, so I hope you've been keeping warm."

Pete was sulking and had begun feverishly wiping his hands on his jacket, so much so that the back of each had begun to bleed.

"I dunno, a day or so I guess. Fuck! I gotta get these cancer cells off of me. I can feel them eating through my flesh."

"Sit up a minute so can look at you. How are you feeling today? Other than the cancer, I mean." Pete sat up and I leaned towards him, studying his face. "You look a little pale."

I placed the back of my hand on Pete's forehead. It was covered in nervous sweat but cool to my touch. "Gosh, Pete, you're burning up," I said.

"Like I'm sick?"

"Yeah. Do you have a sore throat?"

Pete swallowed hard. "Yeah. Sorta."

"Let me take a look." I opened my medical bag and removed a flash light and tongue depressor.

"Open wide and say 'ah.'"

His throat and tonsils looked perfectly normal.

"Hmmmm," I muttered.

"What is it?" Pete asked, his eyes now deep with worry.

"Strep throat!" I tried my damnedest to sound genuinely concerned. "I'm sure of it."

"Oh, GOD!" Pete grunted. He pulled back his head and spit on the ground as if trying to rid the streptococcus from his system.

"Let me feel your neck for swollen glands."

Pete thrust his head forward, turned it side to side so I could examine his neck.

Perfectly normal. "Oh God, Pete, you're loaded with swollen glands."

Tears welled in Pete's eyes and he began to shake. I felt terrible about the charade and taking advantage of his trust. It was betraying everything I believed as a doctor.

"First the cancer and now strep throat," Pete said. "Strep throat can fuck up my heart. I'm no dummy. I know this kinda shit."

"Pete," I said. "All you need is a shot of penicillin and the strep throat will be cured. Just one shot."

He sniffed and tried to gain some composure.

"Really?" Pete said stiffly.

"I guarantee it. Then you can finish your business here in White Mountain and come to Nome for more cancer tests."

He began to relax. He lowered the gun and sat back down on the tundra.

"How do I get a shot of penicillin out here? I can't leave. Too much to do."

"I think I have some right here in my medical bag."

"You're shitting me."

"No, I wouldn't do that, Pete. Give me a minute to check."

Pete laid down the rifle while I rummaged through my bag, searching for a small brown vial I always carried with me. Thorazine.

I found the vial and cradled it in my palm, careful to keep the label out of Pete's view. If he saw it wasn't penicillin, I'd be in serious trouble.

"We're in luck, Pete. I have exactly what we need right here."

I pulled out a syringe and needle and began drawing up some of the yellowish fluid. The dose required to sedate someone of Pete's weight was 50 milligrams—1 cc. But that was the dose to just calm a person down. For my plan to work, Pete needed to be far more than calm. He needed to be out like a light.

I decided 200 milligrams should do the trick. It was a considerable dose and a considerable volume to inject, but I figured I had little to lose. If I didn't give Pete enough to render him unconscious, both he and I would be out of options.

"It goes in your butt so stand up and slip your pants down. No one's looking, so it'll be fine."

Pete stood and edged toward me. He looked suspicious, but I held my composure.

"Ain't you gonna ask me if I'm allergic?" Pete asked. "They do every time they give me a shot."

Shit! Think. Pete's smart and I need to think. If I can't come up with a legitimate answer or I'd be busted!

"It's OK, Pete. I know you're not allergic to penicillin. I remember it from your medical chart."

Pete accepted my answer then slowly lowered his pants to his ankles. Soiled, feces-stained underwear hung loosely around his skinny butt. "Shorts, too," I said.

"I fuckin' hate needles," Pete complained.

"Yeah. Me, too."

He slipped down his undershorts and I was ready to go.

"Now hold still, Pete. This will just take a minute."

I slammed the needle into his buttock and began pumping the potent drug deep into his flesh. He flinched, but I held him firm trying to get the last drop of med to hit its mark.

"Goddammit, that hurts!" Pete cried out. "You're the worst fuckin' shot giver I've ever had."

"Sorry, Pete. I'll be done in a second."

Suddenly Pete lurched and reached behind himself to swat at me. "Take the fuckin' thing out, you're killing me!" Pete screamed. "I'd rather have the strep throat than a goddamn sword sticking me in the ass."

"OK. OK. I'm almost done. You need all the antibiotic to kill the germs."

Finally, the last of the drug was in. I withdrew the needle, capped it, and tossed the setup deep into the guts of my medical bag. I massaged the injection area briskly, hoping it would encourage rapid absorption.

"Son of a fuckin' bitch, I'm never gonna let you give me a shot again!" Pete growled. He drew up a fist as if to slug me, then settled back and reached behind himself to rub his backside.

"I'm sorry, Pete. But trust me. This shot is exactly what you need."

If only he could know how true that is.

Pete pulled up his underwear and pants and sulked back to his rock. He tried to sit, but his ass hurt so much he remained standing.

After a moment, Pete took off his coat, made himself a pillow, and laid down on the soft tundra. I heard him mumble something about taking care of me good if the excruciating penicillin didn't cure his goddamn strep throat.

CHAPTER 57

Twenty minutes dragged by. I sat nervously, waiting for the drug to take effect. Nothing seemed to be happening. Pete's breathing remained regular, and every now and then he mumbled something I wasn't quite able to make out. I started to question if the Thorazine was outdated or if the bottle had somehow been mislabeled.

Thirty minutes passed. Forty. I wondered how long Robert and Darryl's patience would last. About forty-five minutes after I gave the injection, Pete's breathing changed. The whistling became slower and more rhythmic until it softened into a gentle snore. His movements quieted, and he pulled himself up into a fetal position on the cool earth. I walked towards him and looked. Piccolo Pete was asleep.

"Pete?" At first, I whispered, in case he was just snoozing and not unconscious. No response. I called out his name again, louder: "Pete!"

Still no response. I reached down and gently shook his shoulder. He was out cold. I grabbed my stethoscope and blood pressure cuff from my medical bag and checked his vitals. They were all normal.

It worked. Piccolo Pete was completely sedated, immobile yet physically stable. The troops could now be called in and we could head home.

I ran to the top of the ridge and hollered for Robert and Darryl. They rushed over in their ATVs, guns drawn. I told them they could stash their weapons; Pete was under control.

Darryl cuffed Pete and lifted him onto his ATV. We motored back to the landing field, loaded up, and flew back to Nome. Pete whistled in his sleep the entire flight.

Pete was secured overnight in the Nome jail and flown to Anchorage the next day. Once there, I knew he'd be assigned a public defender who would plead insanity, and Pete would end up in a facility for the mentally impaired. It wasn't perfect, but it was better than being buried six feet under the tundra.

Darryl congratulated me on a job well done, and once all official paperwork was executed, he invited me to the BOT to celebrate. I declined, feeling no sense of personal triumph in what I did with Peter Stiles. The fact of the matter was, I felt deeply sad.

I had saved Pete's life. I realized that. But doing it required that I betray his trust, and that went against every personal and professional principle I held sacred. I may have saved Pete's life, but in doing so, I may have left him with little to live for.

CHAPTER 58

I was on a routine radio call to the village of Savoonga on St. Lawrence Island when nurse Connie pounded on the radio room door and rushed in.

"Tom—quick. I need you!"

Connie's voice cracked, and she was visibly shaking. It was panic mode and that got my attention. Connie never panicked.

I signed off the call and chased Connie up the stairs. Bobby Lieberman, a long-time resident of Nome who often worked with Frank, pulled the ambulance up to the hospital's rear doors and jumped out before shutting the ambulance down. I'd only see him do that twice and each time the patient inside had died within moments of arriving. My heart began to flutter.

"What do you have?" I shouted to Bobby. Frank jumped out before Bobby answered, and working together, the two men hauled a gurney out the ambulance rear doors. Both had horrified looks on their faces.

"My God, you won't believe it!" Bobby shouted back. His voice was higher and shakier than usual. "I don't believe it myself."

"Watch the pavement, Doc, it's slippery from last night's rain," Frank said. I saw him reach up with his huge right hand and wipe tears away from his eyes.

I shuffled to the edge of the gurney and pulled back the blanket Bobby had thrown over the patient. Bobby was absolutely right—I could not believe my eyes. It was Gracie.

I gasped, then took Gracie by the shoulders and shook. "Gracie! Wake up!" She did not respond.

"Let's get her in out of the cold," I said. "Connie, get some vitals and grab me a stethoscope."

We inched the gurney through the hospital doors and into the corridor. Once inside Connie ripped open Gracie's nightgown and wrapped a blood pressure cuff firmly around her upper arm.

"What'd you get?"

"Nothing," Connie muttered. "I can't get a blood pressure."

"Try again."

She did.

"Nothing."

"What about pulse?"

"Very weak. Maybe about fifty. So weak I can hardly feel it."

"Get an IV started and draw up an amp of epi while I try to figure out what's happened."

I checked reflexes in Gracie's arms and legs. They were bilaterally unresponsive. I checked the Babinski reflex on both feet. Negative. A good sign. I retracted her upper eyelids and shined a penlight into her pupils. They were pinpoint and sluggishly reactive. It wasn't the best, but better than being fixed and dilated. I called Gracie's name again, but she gave no response. Hating to do it to a friend, I dug a knuckle deep into Gracie's sternum to illicit a pain response. Again, she showed absolutely no reaction.

I glanced over at Bobby and Frank. "Do you have any idea what's going on?"

Frank stepped closer and turned his head for privacy.

"It's her damn ex-boyfriend, Ben Aracutuk," Frank whispered with a trembling voice. "He called me an hour ago and told me to get my black ass over to her house. I asked him why but the SOB hung up without answering. He didn't say it was an emergency and I had a couple of runs to make so I delivered my fares then went over to see her. When I got there and knocked she didn't answer. I was worried, so I opened the door and went inside. That's when I found her lying in her bed. She was in her nightgown so I thought she was sleeping. But when I shook her, and she didn't wake up, I panicked and called Bobby."

"Did you see any blood on her sheets or on her body? Anything unusual?"

Frank shook his head, but Bobby spoke up. "Only this," he said and handed me two brown medicine bottles. "They were sitting on a table right next to her bed along with a half empty glass of water."

One prescription was for INH—isoniazid, a medication used to treat TB. The other was a painkiller, Darvocet. According the bottle labels each prescription had been filled within the past week, yet both bottles were empty. My stomach sank. I was the prescribing physician for both.

Both Frank and Bobby had known Gracie for years. I figured if anyone could answer my next question, it would be one of them.

"You don't think . . . ?"

"I know she's been upset since the last time Ben knocked her around, but I can't believe she would ever hurt herself over it," Bobby said.

"Do either of you know if she's been drinking?"

They both looked away, silent. I had my answer.

Gracie gasped. She arched her back off the table, grunted, then settled back flat and still. The arm holding the blood-pressure cuff went flaccid and the cuff slipped to the floor. A second later, she passed foul smelling gas from her rectum and her head rolled to one side.

Connie shouted, "I don't think she's breathing!"

She was right. Gracie was in respiratory arrest.

CHAPTER 59

I need to intubate her," I barked at Connie. "Get me the laryngoscope and ET tube!"

Connie sped off and grabbed a worn utility cart that Gracie and I had recently converted into an emergency kit. How ironic it was that now, the same cart could be the very key to her survival. Connie drew open the cart's top drawer and searched for the things I needed.

"Got it," Connie said.

"Test the light before you give it to me."

I heard Connie swear under her breath. "No light. Batteries must be dead."

"Get fresh ones. Hurry. I'm going to perform CPR while I wait."

Gracie had a pulse, weak but functional, so she only needed air. I pinched her nose and covered her mouth with mine then began blowing in deep, steady breaths. Her chest rose and fell with my efforts. Success!

Connie returned with the laryngoscope and ET tube. This time, the built-in light worked.

I slipped the endotracheal tube through Gracie's swollen vocal cords and down into her trachea. Then I connected an Ambu breathing bag to the tube and began squeezing.

The bag whistled and wheezed with every pump I gave. Yet, despite its frazzled condition, it worked. I listened with my stethoscope. Enough air was reaching Gracie's lungs to keep her alive until I could figure out what to do next.

I'd been warned about people using a cocktail of INH and Darvocet for suicide attempts, but I'd never seen a case. I knew the overdose was often fatal, and there was no specific treatment except supportive care.

"We can't keep her alive by manual ventilation," I said to Connie. "She needs a ventilator."

"Anchorage?"

"As fast as we can get her there. I'll manage the IVs and bag her. You try to reach Otis and tell him we need the Commander. Tell him it's for Gracie. He knows her."

I knew keeping Gracie alive for a two-hour flight to Anchorage was a long shot, but it was the only option we had for saving her life. Just getting to Anchorage was going to be brutal. The Commander flew half the speed of a jet and to make it over the Alaska Range, we'd have to fly at altitudes so high it would be a challenge to keep her IV running and ventilation going. For the entire trip, I would need to squeeze the Ambu twenty times a minute and, at the same time, monitor her blood pressure and pulse over the noise of the aircraft engines. Should the worst happen and she completely arrest, I'd need to instigate full CPR—a task that would be nearly impossible given our cramped conditions and limited resources.

Ten minutes dragged by while Connie gathered up supplies. My hands started to cramp from squeezing the ventilation bag and my back and shoulders throbbed from leaning forward. I was concerned about how long I could keep the effort up.

We were just about ready to load Gracie back into the ambulance when I had a thought.

"Take over the Ambu for a couple of minutes," I said to Connie. "I need to rest my hands and make a quick call."

Connie grabbed hold of the ventilation bag and went to work. I bolted down the hospital corridor to the telephone.

❖

By the time I returned, Bobby and Frank had finished getting Gracie in the ambulance. I took Frank aside and asked him to do something for me. He nodded and left. Connie handed me the Ambu.

"Let's go," I said to Bobby. "Don't use the siren. I need to be able to hear Gracie's blood pressure and lungs while you drive."

"Hold up a second!" Connie hollered. "Let me get your medical bag. You might need it in flight." She rushed back inside the hospital and returned with my kit.

"Keep in touch, Doc," Connie said. "We all love Gracie. You'll let us know how she's doing?"

I gave Connie a quick hug and smiled. "You know I will."

With that, Bobby slammed the ambulance doors and away we sped.

CHAPTER 60

The twin engines of the 680E Commander aircraft were billowing
foggy mist as Bobby pulled up right along her side.

"How's she doing?" Otis hollered from his open airplane window.

"Not good," I said.

"Does she have an IV running? It makes a difference in my altitude."

"Yes."

"OK. Load her up and I'll get this bird in the air."

A car came screaming up and pulled up next to us. It was Frank's taxi.
Frank slid to a stop and a passenger door flew open. Out popped Pat.

"I'm glad you called," Pat shouted as she ran toward us. "I got Helen and
Don to watch the kids so I could help."

"We'll take turns with the Ambu and checking vitals. I'll manage the IV."

Frank rushed over to help Bobby get Gracie's stretcher into the plane.
I stood by, squeezing the Ambu. As the two were wielding the gurney
through the plane's tight cargo door, something slipped out from under
Gracie's blanket and flittered to the ground. Frank stooped to pick it up.

"It's a note," Frank said. "From Gracie. I recognize her handwriting. It
must have slipped out from her nightgown."

"So, read it, for God's sake," Bobby sputtered. "Hurry."

Frank unfolded the paper and read to himself. He shook his head, looked up at me and frowned as if he didn't fully understand its meaning.

"What's it say, Frank?" I said.

Frank sighed. "She did it . . . with the pills from those bottles. She said it was because of Ben and how he treated her."

"Ah, shit," Bobby said, expressing my sentiments exactly.

Frank began to weep. "That bastard, I could just kill him for this."

I handed Pat the Ambu and went over to put my hand on Frank's shoulder. I knew how much he cared for Gracie. "Enough of that for the moment," I said. "Right now, let's just focus on getting her to Anchorage. She still has a chance to pull through this."

Frank nodded.

"Give me the note," I said. "Could be I'll need it later."

Frank sighed, and with a trembling hand gave me the paper. I absent-mindedly stuffed it away and told Bobby and Frank to get Gracie stabilized for the flight.

Once Gracie's gurney was strapped to the plane's floor, Pat and I climbed aboard. We settled ourselves in the cramped space as comfortably as possible and I checked Gracie's vitals. She hadn't regained consciousness, but her blood pressure and pulse were stable. The problem was she still wasn't breathing on her own.

I whispered a simple prayer of thanks we had Otis at the plane's controls. Three minutes later we were roaring down the runway in a rush of curling wind and pounding rain.

One hour into flight Gracie's IV stopped dripping. I assumed it had either slipped out of the vein and infiltrated into surrounding tissue or was clogged with blood. Whatever the cause, it would be a bitch to fix in the air.

Losing the IV was unacceptable. A running line was the only way to administer emergency drugs should Gracie suffer a heart attack in flight. If that happened, and we had no functioning IV, there would be no defense and Gracie would die.

"Check to see if the IV site is swollen or puffy," I said to Pat. I continued squeezing the Ambu.

Pat had helped me with enough patients to know the signs of a malfunctioning IV. I could rely on her assessment.

"I don't see anything wrong," she said.

"Then maybe it's the altitude. Could be there's not enough pressure at this altitude to keep it running."

I remembered an old trick from med school that helped determine why an IV had stopped running. It wasn't high tech, but it worked.

I removed the IV bottle we'd hung on a stand connected to the gurney and lowered it below Gracie's body. If the line were open, backflow pressure from her venous system would cause blood to seep back up into the IV tubing and we could see it. If I didn't see any blood, it would mean the line was clogged and beyond repair.

I held the bottle in place one second, two, three. Nothing. I lowered the IV further until it was lying on the airplane floor. Then I saw it, a rivulet of blood streaming slowly back into the IV tubing. The IV was open. Low pressure was keeping it from running.

"Can you take us any lower?" I asked Otis. "I think the altitude is affecting Gracie's IV."

Otis shook his head with fervor. "God no! We're already flying lower than we should. Have a look out the window on the left side of the aircraft."

I took my eyes off Gracie long enough to see what Otis meant. Looking out the window, instead of seeing a sky filled with blue sky and clouds, I saw mountaintops and trees *higher* than we were flying, not below us. I understood what Otis was getting at. *We're flying very low, winding our way between the mountain tops, seeking out nooks and crannies to keep our altitude low as possible and still be safe.*

It was not good news. I knew if we stayed at the current altitude much longer, soon Gracie's IV would clog completely shut and stop running. If that happened, all I could do was cling to the hope she wouldn't go into cardiac arrest.

CHAPTER 61

P at looked frightened. "I can't get a blood pressure or pulse," she said. "You try."

She handed me the stethoscope and I listened hard. Nothing.

I twisted myself around in the cramped quarters until I could plant my ear directly over Gracie's chest. I thought perhaps cabin noise and chatter from the plane's radio might be drowning out the sounds of her heartbeat I should hear through the stethoscope. I blocked my free ear with a finger, shut my eyes, and concentrated. I heard nothing but the whishing of air that flowed into her lungs each time Pat squeezed the Ambu.

"She's arrested!" I shouted to Pat. "We've gotta pump her."

I made a fist and punched it onto Gracie's breastbone, hoping the firm thump would jar her heart back into a functional beat. When it didn't, I leaned over and began cardiac compressions. I counted out loud each time I pumped, adjusting my timing to a rate of 100 per minute.

I worked inexhaustibly for ten minutes, stopping every few moments to check her neck and groin for a pulse. Sweat from my brow dripped down onto Gracie's nightgown, soiling it with tiny drops of moisture. I compressed until pain in my back and shoulders forced me to stop to stretch and shake my hands back to life.

She needed intravenous meds, but without a functioning IV there was no way to administer them.

"Grab an amp of adrenaline from my bag," I spluttered to Pat.

Pat rummaged through my medical bag and found what I wanted.

"What kind of needle?"

"Spinal. The longest you can find."

Pat assembled the setup and handed it over.

"Pull open Gracie's nightgown so I can see her chest."

Pat did.

I grasped the needle and syringe in my palm and plunged the needle deep into Gracie's chest. The syringe filled instantly with bright-red blood, meaning I had hit my target. I injected the contents of the syringe directly into Gracie's heart.

Intracardiac adrenaline was our last hope. If the lifesaving med didn't kick-start a heartbeat now, nothing was going to help.

The wait was torturous. I felt every place on Gracie's body where I might perceive a pulse—wrist, groin, neck—but felt nothing. We continued CPR, pausing every few minutes to look and listen for some sign of life. Pat spoke first.

"I think you should check her pupils," Pat whispered.

I looked at Pat with hesitant eyes, not wanting to think what Gracie's pupils might reveal. But I knew she was right. We had allowed more than enough time for the adrenaline work.

I shined a strong beam of light into Gracie's eye. I alternated back and forth, checking repeatedly to be certain my findings were conclusive. No matter how many times I checked, how hard I wanted to see something different, the results remained the same. Gracie's pupils were fully dilated and they failed to react to the light. It was an unmistakable sign of death.

"She's gone, isn't she?" Pat asked.

I nodded.

Pat wiped her eyes and removed the blood pressure cuff from Gracie's arm. I disconnected the Ambu and laid it on the plane's floor.

"Relax your hands and try to stretch your back," I said to Pat. She nodded.

After a few moments I reached down and pulled the now useless breathing tube out of Gracie's mouth. I tossed it on the floor next to the Ambu. Pat covered Gracie's body with a blanket.

Otis needed to know what happened, so I scooted up to the cockpit to tell him. He sighed and shook his head. He told me law required that he radio Anchorage and acknowledge we had a death onboard. I told him I understood, then edged my way back to sit with Pat.

We struggled to keep our gaze away from Gracie and spent the remainder of the flight in absolute silence.

CHAPTER 62

O tis touched the plane down with his signature butter-soft landing and taxied to the terminal for charter aircraft. He braked, but before the engines had completely shut down, two official-looking vehicles approached. The first, a black sedan imprinted with an Alaska State Trooper emblem on the door, came so close I thought it might bump us. The second vehicle, also black and marked with simple block letters—CORONER—pulled in directly behind the first.

A uniformed officer exited the trooper car and motioned for us to deplane. His name tag read Officer William Rice and he did not look like he was in a good mood. I extended my hand to introduce myself. He did not take it.

"You're the PHS physician?" the trooper grumbled.

"I am."

The trooper cocked his head. "Do you have credentials to prove it?"

"Not with me. We've just come in from Nome with a patient who . . ."

"I'm well aware of the purpose of your flight," Officer Rice said coldly. He reached into his coat pocket and removed a notepad and pen.

"What's your name?"

"Is there a problem?"

"I asked your name," the trooper said. "And yes, there's always a problem when someone dies under suspicious circumstances."

I startled. "What do you mean, suspicious circumstances? There's nothing suspicious about what we have here."

"I'll ask a third and last time. Your name—and rank—if you have one?"

"I'm Dr. Thomas J. Sims, Captain with the US Public Health Service, stationed in Nome."

The trooper made some scribbles in his notepad.

"Deceased's name?"

"*The patient's name* is Gracie Kayuk. She is a hospital technician and good friend."

"Presumed cause of death?"

"She took an intentional overdose of INH and Darvocet and went into cardiorespiratory arrest."

"And what makes you think this was a suicide?" The officer kept jotting down things as I spoke.

"We have a note."

The officer nodded. "Show me."

I reached into my jeans pocket and felt around. No note. I checked pockets in my shirt and coat but could not find the goddamn note.

Pat was still sitting in the plane next to Gracie's body. I hollered and asked her if she had the note Frank gave us just before we left.

Pat shook her head. "You stuffed it somewhere."

"Hold on a second," I said to the officer.

I climbed back inside the Commander and searched everywhere I thought the note might have fallen or been placed. I hated to do it, but I even pulled back the blanket covering Gracie's body to check. Nothing.

I explained to the officer the chaos we went through getting Gracie loaded into the plane while intubated, how we struggled to keep her IV running in flight and the intracardiac adrenaline. He seemed satisfied and decided to not hassle us over it any further. I was immensely relieved.

"I'm gonna let it go this time," Officer Rice drawled. "But next time, get yourself more organized or you're gonna find yourself in a heap of trouble."

I wanted to defend our actions further but decided against it. Instead, I just thanked him for the advice.

Officer Rice motioned the coroner over and the two of them worked Gracie's gurney out of the Commander and onto the tarmac. The coroner asked me to step aside until they had finished. When it was time to place her in the hearse, I stepped close to say my goodbyes.

It didn't seem real Gracie was lying there, still and cold beneath a blanket that had started to collect a sprinkling of rain. I took her hand and held it, wondering how I could have failed to see the pain she was suffering so I could help. I felt I had somehow betrayed her, had let her down when she needed me the most. I thought about a time at the BOT when I found her bruised and disheveled but said nothing. I thought about how often she showed up late for work showing signs of trauma and I just let it go. I should have insisted on intervening when I had a chance. I tried, but she resisted. I should have tried harder.

I brushed a clump of hair off Gracie's brow and gazed at her eyes, now closed as if she were sleeping. I searched for answers that didn't come and was left with nothing that gave me comfort.

When I climbed back into the Commander, Pat put her arms around me and kissed me. She was keenly aware of my sense of loss.

Just as the hatch of the plane was about to close, Officer Rice came over and held up a hand.

"Does your chief know you have hair down to your shoulders and you're not wearing a uniform?" the trooper asked.

"I haven't seen my chief since I left Anchorage ten months ago. Why?"

"With your wire rim glasses and hair down to your shoulders, you look more like a goddamn hippie than any PHS physician I've ever seen."

"So the length of my hair and type of glasses I wear are now a crime?" I asked.

The officer shook his head. "Don't be insolent. I'm just saying. Save yourself a lot of grief, Doc. Next time you must deal with authorities, get some real glasses and a haircut to join the club. Life will be a lot easier if you do."

I smiled back at the trooper. "Thanks for the advice, officer, and I'll keep it in mind. It's just that, for the life of me, I've never been much into joining clubs."

We flew home in a somber mood. A few miles out, Otis radioed the Nome tower and asked that Frank be contacted to come meet us at the Munz shack. I was not surprised to see both he and Bobby standing there as Otis pulled the plane up and killed the engines.

We climbed out of the Commander and gave details of what happened. We all hugged and wept.

"I need to get back home," Bobby said. "How about I gather up all the hospital paraphernalia from the plane and bring it over tomorrow?"

I nodded. "Let me get the stuff from my medical bag before you go."

I climbed back into the airplane and scooped up the extra dressings, a few bottles of injectable meds, and some minor instruments scattered around the plane floor. When I tossed them back into my medical bag I noticed something tucked under one of the bag's latches. I used a fingernail to pull it free. It was the suicide note. I'd tossed it in my bag as we were loading Gracie into the plane and had forgotten all about it.

It was one of the toughest days I'd had in Nome, a day that made it clear: life and work in Nome would never be the same again.

CHAPTER 63

Lydia Green was not a happy person.

On the Fourth of July, when we participated in the annual Nome Independence Day Parade by driving the Jeep decorated with flags and the kids tossing candy, Lydia became enraged. Everyone loved us, but Lydia found it distasteful. That day, we laughed with fellow members of the community, ate at the street BBQ, watched the blanket toss, and joined in on all the festivities. We'd been in Nome a year, yet it was the first time we genuinely started to feel part of the Nome community. It was more than Lydia could live with.

Lydia complained bitterly to anyone who would listen about my involvement in civic life. She insisted, because I was a government employee, my family and I were not welcome as true "Nomites." She demanded I resign the position as city health officer I'd been asked to assume because "I was military and had no genuine concern for civic issues." She complained that I operated on animals inside the hospital and disregarded orders from the director of nursing Leona Perone and Harland McCoy, who had become her allies.

The worse accusation of all was that Lydia claimed I provided favored healthcare to the native population of town while ignoring "the whites" because caring for the Eskimos paid my salary. That burned me up to the point of distraction.

Lydia compiled her complaints against me in a scathing letter she mailed to Anchorage. The letter ultimately made it to the office of my commanding officer, Dr. Hayden, and it caused quite a stir.

Two weeks after the July 4 parade, I was summoned to Anchorage to address Lydia's accusations. The meeting would take place in Dr. Hayden's office and would include Lydia Green, Mr. McCoy, Leona Perone, and myself. It would turn out be a meeting that would change everything I believed about my relationship with Nome and the Public Health Service system.

Cold overcast skies matched my mood and created the perfect backdrop for the meeting in Anchorage. We gathered in the waiting area of the commander's office shortly after 8:15 and sat on opposite sides of the room to avoid eye contact. McCoy was dressed in the wrinkled beige suit with matching tie he often wore at work. I had on a simple collared shirt covered by a heavy sweater Pat had knitted and tan slacks. Pat had trimmed my hair to an acceptable PHS length.

I'd never seen Leona dressed in anything but her starched uniform and nursing cap. She looked nice in a dark cotton suit and heels. For a moment, our eyes met and she gave a timid smile that I returned. Lydia Green was in a churchgoing olive green dress that hung well below her knees. She wore her hair in a bun stretched so tightly I wondered if she had trouble blinking. Reading glasses dangled from her neck by a gold chain that caught the lights in the room and projected them into tiny dots across the ceiling.

At 8:30 A.M. sharp, Dr. Hayden's secretary ushered us into her boss's office. Dressed in a decorated dark blue uniform that covered his muscular frame, Dr. Hayden looked every bit the base commander he was. Everyone made proper introductions and Dr. Hayden motioned for us to take seats across from his desk. He started the meeting by warmly addressing me.

"Dr. Sims, it's nice to see you. I don't think we've seen one another since your orientation."

"We haven't, sir," I answered. "It's nice to see you, too. I hope you can come to Nome someday and see what we've accomplished."

I saw McCoy squirm at my remark and heard Lydia Green mutter a disgusted *humph*.

"Did you have something to say, Miss Green?" Dr. Hayden asked. Lydia looked away from the commander's gaze and did not reply.

Dr. Hayden began reading Lydia Green's letter out loud so we could all hear. The room was deadly quiet until the commander set the letter down and began speaking.

"Miss Green," Dr. Hayden began softly. "There are several complaints here, but my staff and I have looked into these thoroughly before this meeting and we have found nothing to substantiate your claims."

Lydia looked up at Dr. Hayden and actually snarled.

"Do you know that Dr. Sims failed to treat a young white boy with a broken arm and his father had to fly the boy to Anchorage in horrible pain to have his arm set?" Lydia asked.

"Miss Green . . . sorry, is it miss or missus?"

"Miss," Lydia said dryly.

"Miss Green. We contacted the father of the boy of whom you speak and learned that is not exactly the case. Dr. Sims was the only physician in town the evening the boy was brought in and he was dealing with two other more emergent situations at the time the boy presented." Dr. Hayden shuffled through a stack of papers and withdrew another letter. He read to himself then spoke again. "According to this letter from the boy's father, his son was given pain medication, X-rays were taken, his wound was scrubbed, and he was given a temporary splint while Dr. Sims was dealing with other, more serious emergencies. It wasn't until Dr. Sims came looking for the boy that he learned the father had come and collected his son. So, Dr. Sims was never able to *treat* the boy because the boy was gone before he had an opportunity to get to him."

Lydia shuffled in her seat. "Well that's not the way I heard it!" she growled.

Dr. Hayden continued. "Actually, the boy's father apologized for the way he acted. He was just worried about his son and didn't stop to think the entire situation through."

Lydia huffed and looked towards McCoy and Leona. Neither met her gaze.

"Now I'd like to address the complaint about Dr. Sims taking care of animals in the hospital," Dr. Hayden added.

"Please do," Lydia said.

Dr. Hayden picked up two more letters and began to read.

"I have several letters from members of the Nome community—both the Caucasian and native populations I might add. These letters express overwhelming gratitude to Dr. Sims for taking care of their sick and injured pets."

"Yes! But right in the hospital and against Leona's rule?"

"Dr. Sims has taken care of many animals—mostly dogs—right in his home. There was only one occasion when a dog, belonging to a tourist, was so severely injured that Dr. Sims needed instruments available only at the hospital. In that circumstance Dr. Sims did *not* use the operating room as you stated in your letter. He used a patient room that was thoroughly cleaned and disinfected after he operated and saved the little dog's life."

"This meeting is fixed!" Lydia shouted and bolted out of her chair. She turned to head for the door when Dr. Hayden said in his most authoritative voice, "Take your seat, Miss Green. These allegations are very serious, and we will take care of them right now."

Lydia seethed, but sat back down as Dr. Hayden commanded.

Dr. Hayden then turned his attention to the hospital administrator. "Mr. McCoy, Miss Green claims you were never paid by the owner of the dog who was operated on inside the hospital. Is that true?"

McCoy's lower lip began to tremble. "At first, yes," he muttered.

"But then?"

"OK. Later we contacted the charter outfit in Anchorage who brought the hunters up to Nome to hunt polar bears. We got in touch with the people and sent them an invoice."

"And did they pay?"

"Finally."

"And did you give some of that payment to Dr. Sims?"

McCoy paused. The tremor on his lower lip heightened. Clearly, he hated to answer the question. Finally, he said, "We did not."

"And why didn't you? Wasn't it Dr. Sims who saved the dog's life? Didn't you think he was entitled to some compensation for what he did?"

McCoy paused again to consider his answer. "We felt Dr. Sims was responsible for collecting his own fee."

"And did you provide Dr. Sims with the contact information you were able to obtain about the person?"

McCoy did not answer.

"Dr. Sims, did you receive any compensation from the dog owners or the hospital for your services?"

"No, sir."

"Did you receive any information about the people so you could send them your own fees?"

"No, sir."

"One more thing, Mr. McCoy." He glanced down at other paperwork in his hands. "Am I to understand you sent Dr. Sims a bill for the delivery of his own son? Is that correct?"

I could hardly wait to hear McCoy's answer.

"Yes," the administrator whispered.

"Could you speak up, sir? I can barely hear you."

"Yes, that's true. We did send Dr. Sims a bill."

"And did that bill include a charge for . . . let me see how you worded it . . . physician services?"

McCoy whimpered again. "It did."

"Sir?"

"It did, yes," McCoy said louder.

"And do you understand the 'physician services' you billed were for work Dr. Sims *himself* did when he delivered his own son? Is that right?"

"Sort of."

"Sort of, Mr. McCoy? That is your answer?"

At that Dr. Hayden stood and looked the administrator squarely in the eyes. "You, sir, specifically tried to defraud Dr. Sims and the United States government. I suggest you go back to your hospital and thoroughly read the contract the US Public Health Service has with your institution. I also suggest you take extreme caution when dealing with Dr. Sims or any other member of the PHS from here on out, or you and your hospital will find yourself embroiled in politics, audits, and legal maneuvers you do not want to be a party to."

McCoy sat quietly and perfectly still except for the repeated swallowing he didn't seem able to control.

"Do I make myself clear?" Dr. Hayden asked forcefully.

"Perfectly," McCoy answered.

Dr. Hayden then sat back down and turned his attention to Leona.

"Miss Perone, I understand you are the director of nursing at the hospital. Is that correct?"

Leona answered with a mouth so dry she could barely speak. "Yes, sir. That is correct."

"Do you believe that position also authorizes you as Dr. Sims's director?"

Leona stared at the floor and did not answer the question.

"Allow me to remind you, Miss Perone, that Dr. Sims is an officer in the United States Public Health Service. He works under a very, very specific government contract the United States government has with the MMM Hospital. That means he reports and takes orders directly from me and this office and no one else. That includes you, madam."

Leona lowered her head but said nothing.

"If you do not understand this contractual agreement I recommend you hastily learn about it from your director, Mr. McCoy, and that you do so before offering up any further complaints about the physician you are expected to assist."

Leona sighed.

"Do you understand, madam? Do you have any questions?"

Leona shook her head but did not speak.

Dr. Hayden took a deep breath then addressed the entire group.

"As for Dr. Sims and his family becoming a part of the Nome community, I have to say I am ashamed of all of you for taking offense at this. You should be proud of what he has accomplished in just one year. From what I have learned from his superiors at the Kotzebue Service Unit, the village health aides he works with seven days a week, and members of the community Dr. Sims has done a remarkable job of bringing the Public Health Service's system of healthcare to all the people of the area—native and nonnative alike. He is respected and well liked. He and his wife even had their son in Nome. That's something we rarely, if ever, see in one of our physicians serving in remote areas."

I was speechless, as were Lydia Green, McCoy, and Leona Perone.

Dr. Hayden continued, "If there are no further questions or comments, this meeting is adjourned. Mr. McCoy, Miss Green, Miss Perone, please see yourselves out. Dr. Sims, will you please stay a moment longer?"

I was overwhelmed by what had happened. Dr. Hayden and I spent the next thirty minutes discussing how difficult life and work had become in Nome. I told him about the struggles I initially encountered because of what happened with my predecessor. I told him how malignant the relationship had become between the MMM Hospital and myself and how McCoy and Leona tried to sabotage every effort I made to bring our two systems of healthcare together.

"I'm aware Nome is complicated. It always has been. But you've been in Nome a year now and you have one more to go. What are your thoughts about getting through this and moving forward?"

It was a question I wasn't expecting. "I'm not sure," I said after a beat. "I doubt much will change, even after a meeting like this."

Dr. Hayden nodded. "I suspect you're right. So, what do you think you want to do?"

The question caught me off guard, especially since I didn't know I had any say on where I wanted to go or do. "May I get back to you on that?" I asked.

Dr. Hayden stood and extended his hand. "Of course. Just let me know what you think."

I shook Dr. Hayden's hand, thanked him for being so supportive in the meeting, and left his office. That afternoon I boarded the same plane as Lydia, McCoy, and Leona for the flight back to Nome. They sat together several rows behind me, yet I swore I could feel hostility oozing from their pores.

When I got home I gave Pat all the details of the meeting and the conversation afterward with Dr. Hayden. I told her I wasn't sure what the commander meant when he asked for my thoughts about moving forward. Was he hinting I might be leaving Nome for another location?

If he was, could I honestly provide any input as to where I wanted to be stationed?

I felt validated by Dr. Hayden's encouraging words, but it wasn't enough. If there was even the slightest chance a reassignment of duty might be possible it was something Pat and I needed to discuss at length. And that is what we did for the rest of the night.

The following morning, I took out a pad and pen and wrote Dr. Hayden a letter requesting a transfer out of Nome.

CHAPTER 64

We were excited about celebrating Adam's first birthday. Pat planned a party with gifts, cake, ice cream and snacks, all the things we couldn't afford but prioritized anyway. My prayer was that the party would turn out better than the one we tried for his first Christmas.

We were set for 2:00. The phone rang at 1:30.

"Tom, it's Dave."

Dave Higgins was a doctor that occasionally came down from Kotzebue to help cover Nome. We worked well together, and it was always a relief when he was in town. He was going to cover calls so I could have a much-needed day off and enjoy my boy's first birthday.

"What's up?"

"Bad news. I've got a burn in Golovin I need to go out and check. Problem is, I've also got a guy with a stab wound coming in from St. Michaels. I hate to do this to you, with the party and all, but I need you to check on the stabbing when it comes in."

Crap! It never ends.

"Is the stabbing victim stable?"

"Village health aide thinks so. I guess he's drunk, but vitals are fine."

"OK. Adam's party starts in half an hour," I told Dave. "Ask Barbara to give me a call when he arrives."

"You got it," Dave said. "Remember, Barbara's still a little green."

"I remember. Please let me know when you get back from Golovin."

"I will."

At precisely two o'clock the doorbell rang, and everyone shuffled in. Jamie and Billy came with a toy pickup truck I'd seen at the NC. Esther came with a pair of handmade tiny mukluks. Several nurses from the hospital and DJs from KNOM were there, all bearing gifts and appetites. Helen and Don had stuffed a large plastic trash bag full of balloons elaborately painted with colorful faces of clowns and animals. Adam loved their gift the most, and immediately began laughing and batting at the colorful balloons as Don played catch and peekaboo with him.

At 3:15 Barbara called. She told me to hustle up to the hospital immediately. She felt the stabbing victim did not look good.

I estimated the patient's age at mid-twenties, but it was hard to tell since his face was covered in grime and he was too intoxicated to answer questions. He was lying face up on a gurney, shirtless and covered by a blood-soiled wool blanket. Barbara gave me his vitals. They were stable.

Most doctors, myself included, dislike evaluating drunken patients. They usually smell, are belligerent, uncooperative, and frequently aggressive.

"Goddammit!" the man said, swinging his fist toward my face when I tried lifting the blanket covering him. "Get the fuck away from me."

I jumped back, then grabbed his arm and shoved it against his side. I resisted the temptation to punch him. I snatched up a portion of the gurney sheet, wrapped it around his assertive arm and tucked it under his hip to restrain it.

"You smack me again and I'll throw you out of this hospital," I said to the kid. "Now settle down and shut up."

"He smacked at me, too, when I tried lifting the blanket," Barbara said. "That's when I called you."

I looked down at the patient and tried to engage his eyes.

"We're just trying to help you," I said. "What's your name?"

"Charles," he muttered, and after a moment's pause added, "Charlie."

"OK, Charlie. You're in Nome Hospital and I'm Dr. Sims. Can you tell me what happened?"

"They hit me . . . the motherfuckers pulled a knife . . ." Charlie began to whimper.

"I need to pull this blanket back and see your belly."

Charlie wildly shook his head, spraying saliva about the room. "No, Doc. It kills me when someone touches the blanket."

"OK," I said. "Let me give you something for pain first."

Vital signs were stable, so I asked Barbara to give him a shot of Demerol and Phenergan and start an IV.

The pain shot, potentiated by the booze, took effect in less than ten minutes. When Charlie was snoring peacefully, I lifted one edge of the blanket and had a look. It was bad.

A deep, ten-inch stab wound ran across the upper portion of Charlie's abdomen. Protruding from the wound, curled like a rattlesnake ready to strike, lay a length of small intestines two feet long. Blood from the wound had pooled around the glob of intestines then dried, adhering his guts to the underside of the blanket covering him. Every time the blanket was moved, Charlie's intestines were pulled out from his abdominal cavity.

Charlie was in no immediate danger, but a deep stab wound to the abdomen required prompt abdominal exploration. It was a surgical emergency I wasn't equipped to handle.

"Call Munz and order a charter to Anchorage," I said to Barbara. "Tell them we have a patient on a stretcher with IV running and he'll have escorts."

"Otis?"

"If he's available. If not, Sparky O'Neil."

"You got it, boss."

I needed to talk with Dave. I radioed Munz and had them patch me through to his charter. They were still in flight so I reached him on the first try. I told Dave what I had going on and when he thought he'd be back in Nome.

The connection was broken up with static, but I heard enough to understand him say he'd be back in Nome in less than an hour.

It was what I was hoping to hear.

Hot damn! The day was looking up.

"Dave, I need to accompany this guy to Anchorage so I'm going to be leaving. I'll have Barbara keep an eye on the hospital till you get back. She should be fine for just an hour."

4:15 P.M.

Pat answered on the third ring.

"How's the party going?"

"Everyone left shortly after you went to the hospital. But it's OK. Chantelle and Adam are tired, so I put them down for a nap."

"What do you think about waking the kids up and coming with me to Anchorage? I have a charter and the plane's big enough for us all."

I didn't need to wait for her answer.

Charlie arrived without problems and we whisked him off to surgery. I scrubbed in on the case and saw firsthand my instincts were right. This *was* a surgical emergency. The knife had punctured a hole in the colon that, had it not been discovered, would have led to peritonitis and death.

Dr. Hurlbert, the surgeon on the case, patted me on the back after we closed Charlie up and removed our surgical gowns. "Your training must have been good. You saved this guy's life."

I accepted the compliment with pleasure. There had been so few of them since I'd arrived in Nome. "Thanks," I said, then went to the doctor's lounge to change back into my street clothes. I was anxious to meet up with my family and have a night on the town.

We stayed in Anchorage three days and it was just the break Pat needed. I rented a car and we went out to a real restaurant. We gathered around the table laughing and enjoying a dinner of pizza, beer, real milk, and baby formula. We mused over where life had taken us. The next day I took Pat shopping—real shopping—in stores where choices weren't limited to basics and prices were in a range we could afford. Pat loved the freedom and conveniences the city gave her—grocery stores with fruits and vegetables, fresh meat, eggs and milk; lights that worked most of the time; flush toilets and running water that didn't come from a tank. I could read her mind: she was tiring of life in the Arctic frontier.

CHAPTER 65

The ambulance tore into the emergency area with siren blaring. I knew it was a bad sign. Bobby hopped out with a look on his face I hadn't seen since the day he brought in Gracie.

I ran out to help and asked Bobby what he had. He was too choked up to answer. Instead, he pointed to his gurney that held a very large person completely covered by a blanket.

"I'm afraid it's not an ambulance this trip," Bobby managed to say. "I'm afraid it's a hearse."

A chill like electric current shot through my body. We pulled the gurney out of the ambulance and I lifted the blanket. My eyes glazed over when I looked down and saw a swollen face I had grown to trust and adore.

"Oh God, no!" I muttered. It was Frank.

Bobby started to speak but I stopped him with a rise of my hand. I wanted to check to see if there was anything we could do for our friend.

I placed my stethoscope over Frank's huge chest and listen for a heartbeat. It was out of habit, not necessity. Frank's skin was already mottled

295

and corpselike—cold to my touch and stiff. Both pupils were fixed and dilated. Any benefits of CPR had long passed.

"Do you know what in God's name happened?" I asked Bobby.

Bobby, barely able to speak, gave me as much history as he had. "Frank's neighbors, Jack and Betty Johnson, invited him to their place for a fried chicken dinner. They knew he was still mourning Gracie's passing. They were eating when Frank said he didn't feel well and had to go to the bathroom. When he didn't come back to the table, Jack went to check and found him lying on the floor. Jack shook him, but when he didn't respond they called me. I rushed right over and found him like this."

I shook my head. "How long ago was that?"

"A good thirty minutes now. Maybe more. I thumped on his chest like I'd seen you do, and even blew air into the lungs, but it didn't help."

The hospital door flew open and Helen came out. When she saw what had happened, she gasped and drew her hand up to her face in disbelief.

We stood around Frank's lifeless form lost for words. How could life be so normal one moment then become so drastically different the next?

With nothing to be done, Bobby and I loaded Frank's body back into the ambulance for his final trip, this one to the city morgue.

Frank was overweight. He had high blood pressure and diabetes. He probably suffered a heart attack, but we'd never know for sure. Bobby fretted over wondering if he could have done more for him before hauling him in. I assured him that wasn't the case; Frank was gone before he ever got to him.

Nome's city morgue was nothing more than a small wooden shack built on a hill just outside of town. It was used for storage, a macabre place where bodies were kept frozen all winter long until summer thaw allowed the ground to be dug for burials. It was empty now, as burials for the year had been completed.

I found some peace knowing Frank would not be kept in the morgue, wrapped in a plastic bag waiting to be interred. His burial would be done the next day to a sizable crowd sad to see his passing. But the peace wasn't enough to ease my pain. Losing Frank was a blow I wasn't prepared to handle.

I hadn't heard from Dr. Hayden about the letter I'd written requesting a transfer out of Nome, so I began writing again. I wrote every week. After seeing Pat's joy on our recent trip to Anchorage, I no longer wanted a different assignment in the bush. I wanted us to go to Anchorage, the big city with conveniences and a place where I could blend in with the masses and feel less emotionally connected to people who depended on me for life and death decisions. I wanted freedom from the hostile environment of Nome that polarized the community against me and the work I was trying to do. And I was sick of the archaic conditions with no reasonable help or support. Worst of all, winter was coming and I loathed the thought of living again in darkness.

I had reached the bleakest moment of my experience in the Arctic and now, all I wanted to do was escape.

CHAPTER 66

T he letter came in a windowed envelope designated "Official Government Use Only." For an instant, my mind raced back to a letter I'd received years before from Creighton University, and how one simple page had changed the direction my life would take. I held my breath as I opened and read from a sheet of letterhead paper, wondering if the same were about to happen.

A position had opened in the department of obstetrics and gynecology at the Alaska Native Medical Center in Anchorage. I had been approved to fill it. A written response was requested within forty-eight hours and the transfer, should I decide to accept it, would take place in just two weeks. The letter was signed by Dr. William Hayden, Base Commander, United States Public Health Service, Anchorage, Alaska.

I rushed home after clinic to show the letter to Pat. We sat down in the living room for a serious discussion.

"Is it what you want?" Pat said.

I paused. "A month ago I thought it was. You?"

"I'll always be in your corner wherever you want to go."

"We have friends here," I said.

"We'll make new ones in Anchorage."

OB-GYN wasn't my first choice, but Anchorage was. Given the experience I'd gained doing deliveries in the Arctic, I felt I could do a good job in the position.

Closing out my work in Nome, packing up our belongings, and saying goodbye to loyal friends would be a major change in our lives. If we decided yes, it would be permanent and happen sooner than we thought.

"So, what do you think I should do?" I asked.

Pat smiled and handed me a paper and pen.

Pat was ready for movers the morning they arrived two weeks later. Food, dishes, clothing, and what few personal items we had were packed in boxes and taped shut. PHS would have them picked up the next day and flown to Anchorage. Dave was going to cover Nome until permanent arrangements for another full-time doctor could be made so I spent most of my time bringing him up to speed on issues I thought required his attention.

The Pontiac presented a problem. PHS regulations required that, whenever an officer was transferred to a different post, vehicles had to be shipped by *surface* transportation. I argued the point with headquarters in Anchorage since there were no roads, trains, or other means of ground connection between Anchorage and Nome except the ocean and sending the car by sea would take months for it to arrive. Sadly, no exceptions could be made.

We would need our car immediately in Anchorage, so our only choice was to pay Alaska Airlines $200 ourselves to fly the station wagon and get it there in an hour. I could live with that major hit to our personal budget, but only if I could get maximum benefit from its spoils. I came up with an idea.

"Can you give me a hand here?" I asked one of the moving guys after Pat had given them a cup of coffee during a break.

"Sure," the fellow said. "What do you need?"

"This."

I pointed to our Yamaha motorcycle and asked him to help me load it into the back of the Pontiac. It was a tight fit, but we got it in.

"Pack all your house plants, tomatoes, potted herbs, even the tropical fish inside the car," I said to Pat. She had decided to give the fish away and toss all the plants because we couldn't carry them on the plane. "Stuff everything close together so nothing will tip over and leave just enough room for me to squeeze behind the wheel."

Pat did as I asked. When she finished, I called Jamie and Billy and asked them to pick up Pat and the kids and follow me to the airport.

"What about da snowmachine?" Billy asked when he pulled his truck up close to the Pontiac so we could talk.

"I have some guys coming back later today to crate it up. They'll take it to the dock where it will be loaded on the next barge."

"You payin' to ship it to Anchorage?"

I shook my head. "Nope, the PHS is. Technically it's a vehicle, so PHS will transport it. Since we won't be needing it in Anchorage, I'll sell it. It'll take a while to arrive since it must go by barge, but I don't care. It'll be winter when it gets there, and we'll get a better price there than we would in Nome. Probably more than the $200 I'm paying to fly the car."

Billy grinned. "You sly devil, you always t'inking," he said, smiling through those snow-white teeth of his.

I asked Pat to come stand by me for one last look at the trailer that had been our Arctic home for the last ten months. We wrapped our arms around each other and I heard Pat sigh. Strong, emotion-packed memories flooded over us as we reminisced about the life we were leaving behind. Sadness, mixed with joy, filled our hearts.

"The plane's due soon," Billy shouted from his pickup window. "We should head out now."

I helped Pat get herself and the kids into Billy's truck then tucked myself behind the wheel of our overstuffed car. I drove a little slower than usual, to savor the moment. I wished there had been room in the Pontiac for Pat to join me for that one last drive away from home.

CHAPTER 67

I wanted to ease out of town; say goodbye to a few key people then fade away with no more fanfare than when we came in. Billy and Jamie would have none of that.

We pulled up in front of the Alaska Airlines terminal to a blaze of people. Music blared from speakers set up outside and folks were milling about laughing, dancing, and downing beer and wine like it was free because it was. A banner had been hung over a table loaded with cake, ice cream and coffee that read: "Goodbye and Best of Luck Dr. and Mrs. Sims. We will miss you." It was a send-off that tore at my heartstrings.

Jim Weston, owner of the BOT, had graciously provided free hors d'oeuvres and all manner of spirits anyone could want. Clara, my favorite server at the BOT, was having a great time pouring beverages. McCoy was there with his wife, making congratulatory speeches mostly directed toward himself, as if all the medical work accomplished in Nome was of his doing. Dave was there as were Helen and Don, Billy and Jamie, Father Poole from KNOM radio, and the rest of the hospital gang who made our lives livable. Connie began to cry when we talked about our night together trying to save the boy who inhaled glue but also her joy in being present at the birth of our son. Helen and Don couldn't help but reminisce about the snowmachine accident that sent Adam leaving a bloody trail across a frozen path. The only person from the hospital not in attendance was Leona Perone; her absence explained by McCoy who said she stayed on duty so other nurses, who knew me better, could attend the party and see us off.

Mary and David Torrington owned a gift shop in town and shortly after arriving in Nome, I delivered their baby. They presented us with a beautiful ivory carving we had admired but couldn't afford. Ed Greenberg, my seal-hunting buddy, gifted us with a bottle of Crown Royal.

An hour shot by and our flight was announced. I turned to Esther and Bobby. Other than Billy and Jamie, I would miss them the most.

"So, young doctor, you gonna give dis ole Eskimo woman a hug afore you leave?" Esther asked. She spoke with raw emotion I'd never heard from an Eskimo woman and I caught an unmistakable glimmer in her eyes.

"Get over here!" I drawled and threw my arms around her to draw her close. "You've been a wonderful assistant and a great friend. I will miss you more than you will ever know."

Esther loosened our embrace and gently took my face in her hands.

"You been da best and kindest doctor Nome ever see," she muttered. "It has been my great joy to work for you."

"*With* me." I said. And Esther smiled.

Then Bobby came up and poured his arms around me.

"Goodbye, Doc." Bobby said. "It's been really great getting to know you." He began to weep, and I knew his tears were as much for Frank as they were for my departure.

I felt a tap on my shoulder. It was Allison Brown, the airline receptionist.

"I'm sorry, Dr. Sims, but you and the family need to get on board the aircraft. It's time to leave."

She couldn't have said it better. It *was* time to leave Nome. It had *been* time for quite a while.

We boarded the jet and settled into our seats. Pat chose the window and kept Adam on her lap. I sat on the aisle with Chantelle nestled between us. The engines roared to life and moments later we soared into a cloudless sky.

"There she goes," Pat said as she gazed out the window and watched our little coastal town fade in the distance.

"You OK?" I asked.

She turned to me and smiled. "I'm fine. It's just that we're leaving a segment of our life and people I care about. But I'm happy we're going. I'm looking forward to the change." She paused. "I'm also happy I got to share this adventure with you."

I took Pat's hand in mine and kissed it. I held it tightly for the next several minutes but had nothing more to say. I knew many emotions filled her heart and felt it best to let them linger as long as she wanted.

When it began, life in the Arctic shattered our world. It was a journey for which we had no training, no experience, and no desire to embrace. For sixteen months, I emptied my heart and soul into the Nome community; many times feeling I received nothing in return but heartache and grief. But by the time we left, our journey in the bush had become something quite different.

I closed my eyes and allowed my thoughts to drift back to the adventures I'd lived and medical feats I'd conquered. I thought about babies I'd delivered, my own son's birth, surgeries I'd performed and risks I'd taken. I thought about Piccolo Pete and hoped, one day, he'd forgive me for the actions I took to save his life. And I thought about Gracie and Frank, the pain of losing them, and how their deaths had had such an impact on our hospital family.

No amount of preparation could have readied me for what I faced in the Arctic. It was only by living the adventure, making mistakes, relying on my instincts and relentlessly hunting for solutions that I could have found my way.

I came to Nome a young physician, full of enthusiasm but laden with self-doubt. I left a better man, a better husband and father, and a better doctor. Life and work in Nome had shown me a roadmap for my life that would guide me into the future. And as I, like my wife, peered out the aircraft window and watched Nome fade away, I realized in so many ways *Nome had given far more to me than I had ever given her back in return.*

EPILOGUE

L ife changed after we moved to Anchorage, very much like we knew it would. The OB-GYN department was small and I liked that. My immediate chief was Dr. John Macintosh, the same jerk who hung up on me when I frantically called that night for advice on how to handle Juliette's shoulder presentation. At first, working with him because of that took some attitude adjustment on my part, but I quickly learned to live with it and moved on.

John ran the department smoothly and he made me feel welcomed as part of the team. We worked well together on difficult deliveries and complicated surgeries, and I learned a great deal from him about obstetrics that I took into my private practice after leaving the PHS. One night over dinner at his house accompanied by a couple of glasses of wine, I brought up my call about the shoulder presentation. He claimed he didn't recall the case.

We had a second general medical officer (GMO) like myself on our service, Dr. Parker Smith. Before coming to Anchorage, Parker had never set foot in a town smaller than five hundred thousand people and to him, being confined to a city the size of Anchorage was like living in the sticks. Parker enjoyed life smooth and easy. He made it very clear he would never, under any circumstances, go out to the bush on a temporary duty assignment (TDY) to care of problems even if his commission in the PHS required him to do so. Instead, he insisted I keep my go-bag stocked and ready to go because if a call for TDY ever came to OB-GYN, that call would always go to me.

We had a civilian midwife, Ingrid Gustafson, working with us. Ingrid made my life perfect. She handled most of the daytime deliveries and rotated night and weekend call with the rest of us on the team. Basically, I was on-call only one weekend per month. Easy-peasy.

We formed new friendships in Anchorage, none as strong or binding as the relationships we enjoyed in Nome, but enough to satisfy our need for social interaction.

The biggest change that came after leaving the Arctic was with our family life. I no longer suffered the burden of being available every minute of every day. Rather, it felt like I was on an extended vacation. I showed up for work around 8:00 A.M., made rounds on what few patients I had in the hospital, then simply hung around for surgeries that might or might not materialize during the day. Outpatient clinic began daily at 1:30 and ended at 4:30 sharp. I always got home before dinner and rarely was called out at night for an emergency.

I was also bored out of my mind.

The boredom didn't last. During the eight months I was stationed in Anchorage, I was the most experienced physician at the hospital accustomed to practicing frontier medicine in the bush. Because of that I was frequently asked to take TDY assignments in remote areas all around the state. I had the opportunity to travel most of Alaska, meet more people, and have more adventures than anyone else I knew in the Service.

My final months in Alaska rekindled my love of medicine, something I feared I'd lost in Nome. After a while, I discovered it wasn't *medical* practice that pushed me from the bush, it was politics and conflicts that had nothing to do with the reason I became a physician in the first place.

Pat and I never returned to Nome, but thoughts of our friends, coworkers, and the experiences we had there have lived on in our memories and have shaped our lives. We eventually settled in a small town in rural Oregon where, once again, we could become part of a community and I could rekindle my joy of being a family doctor. The land was magnificent, the people devine, and the air could not be seen, smelled, or tasted.

I have more stories to tell of those marvelous years in Oregon, stories I'd love to share in another book. All I need is for a friend to sit with me in a local pub, raise a glass of Crown Royal, listen hard and tell me: "Drink up, Doc. I've got all night."